15,~

The Secret of Yoga

RELIGIOUS PERSPECTIVES · VOLUME TWENTY-THREE

The Secret of Yoga

GOPI KRISHNA

1817

HARPER & ROW, PUBLISHERS

NEW YORK, EVANSTON, SAN FRANCISCO, LONDON

RELIGIOUS PERSPECTIVES

VOLUMES ALREADY PUBLISHED

Contents

Religious Perspectives

Its Meaning and Purpose

Religious perspectives represents a quest for the rediscovery of man. It constitutes an effort to define man's search for the essence of being in order that he may have a knowledge of goals. It is an endeavor to show that there is no possibility of achieving an understanding of man's total nature on the basis of phenomena known by the analytical method alone. It hopes to point to the false antinomy between revelation and reason, faith and knowledge, grace and nature, courage and anxiety. Mathematics, physics, philosophy, biology, and religion, in spite of their almost complete independence, have begun to sense their interrelatedness and to become aware of that mode of cognition which teaches that "the light is not without but within me, and I myself am the light."

My Introduction to this Series is not of course to be construed as a prefatory essay for each individual book. These few pages simply attempt to set forth the general aim and purpose of the Series as a whole. They try to point to the humanistic and transcendent significance of the creative process in the respective disciplines as represented by those scholars who have been invited to participate in this endeavor.

Modern man is threatened by a world created by himself. He

is faced with the conversion of mind to naturalism, a dogmatic secularism and an opposition to a belief in the transcendent. He begins to see, however, that the universe is given not as one existing and one perceived but as the unity of subject and object; that the barrier between them cannot be said to have been dissolved as the result of recent experience in the physical sciences, since this barrier has never existed. Confronted with the question of meaning, he is summoned to rediscover and scrutinize the immutable and the permanent which constitute the dynamic, unifying aspect of life as well as the principle of differentiation; to reconcile identity and diversity, immutability and unrest. He begins to recognize that just as every person descends by his particular path, so he is able to ascend, and this ascent aims at a return to the source of creation, an inward home from which he has become estranged.

It is the hope of RELIGIOUS PERSPECTIVES that the rediscovery of man will point the way to the rediscovery of God. To this end a rediscovery of first principles should constitute part of the quest. These principles, not to be superseded by new discoveries, are not those of historical worlds that come to be and perish. They are to be sought in the heart and spirit of man, and no interpretation of a merely historical or scientific universe can guide the search. RELIGIOUS PERSPECTIVES attempts not only to ask dispassionately what the nature of God is, but also to restore to human life at least the hypothesis of God and the symbols that relate to him. It endeavors to show that man is faced with the metaphysical question of the truth of religion while he encounters the empirical question of its effects on the life of humanity and its meaning for society. Religion is here distinguished from theology and its doctrinal forms and is intended to denote the feelings, aspirations, and acts of men, as they relate to total reality. For we are all in search of reality, of a reality which is there whether we know it or not; and the search is of our own making but reality is not.

RELIGIOUS PERSPECTIVES is nourished by the spiritual and intellectual energy of world thought, by those religious and ethical leaders who are not merely spectators but scholars deeply involved in the critical problems common to all religions. These thinkers recognize that human morality and human ideals thrive only when set in a context of a transcendent attitude toward religion and that by pointing to the ground of identity and the common nature of being in the religious experience of man, the essential nature of religion may be defined. Thus, they are committed to reevaluate the meaning of everlastingness, an experience which has been lost and which is the content of that *visio Dei* constituting the structure of all religions. It is the many absorbed everlastingly into the ultimate unity, a unity subsuming what Whitehead calls the fluency of God and the everlastingness of passing experience.

The false dichotomies, created by man, especially Western man, do not exist in nature. Antinomies are unknown in the realm of nature. The new topology of the earth implies the link between an act and a whole series of consequences; and a consciousness of the individual that every time a decision is made it has distant consequences which become more precisely determined.

Furthermore, man has a desire for "elsewhere," a third dimension which cannot be found on earth and yet which must be experienced on earth: prediction: detailed statement referring to something that is to happen in the future; projection: combining a number of trends; prevision: that which is scientifically probable and likely to happen; prospective: the relation between present activity and the image of the future; plan: the sum of total decisions for coordinated activities with a goal in mind.

The authors in RELIGIOUS PERSPECTIVES attempt to show that to *be* is more important than to have since *being* leads to transcendence and joy, while having only leads to apathy and despair.

Man has now reached the point of controlling those forces both outside himself and within himself which throughout history hemmed in decision-making. And what is decisive is that this new trend is irreversible. We have eaten of this new tree of knowledge and what fifty years ago seemed *fate* has now become the subject of our deliberate choices. Therefore, for man, both in the East and in the West, the two basic questions are: What proper use can we make of our knowledge both for the spirit and for the body and what are the criteria for our choices? Only the answers to these questions, which conform to the new reality, can assure the continuity of human life and preserve the human person who is related not only to the present but also to the past and therefore to the future in a meaningful existence. The choice is ours.

These volumes seek to show that the unity of which we speak consists in a certitude emanating from the nature of man who seeks God and the nature of God who seeks man. Such certitude bathes in an intuitive act of cognition, participating in the divine essence and is related to the natural spirituality of intelligence. This is not by any means to say that there is an equivalence of all faiths in the traditional religions of human history. It is, however, to emphasize the distinction between the spiritual and the temporal which all religions acknowledge. For duration of thought is composed of instants superior to time, and is an intuition of the permanence of existence and its meta-historical reality. In fact, the symbol[1] itself found on cover and jacket of each volume of RELIGIOUS PERSPECTIVES is the visible sign or representation of the essence, immediacy, and timelessness of religious experience; the one immutable center, which may be analogically related to being in pure act, moving with centrifugal and ecumenical necessity outward into the manifold modes, yet simultaneously, with dynamic centripetal power and with full intentional energy, returning to the source. Through the very diversity of its authors, the Series shows that the basic and poignant concern of every faith is to point to, and overcome the crisis in our apocalyptic epoch—the crisis of man's separation from man and of man's separation from God—the failure of love. The

[1] From the original design by Leo Katz.

authors endeavor, moreover, to illustrate the truth that the human heart is able, and even yearns, to go to the very lengths of God; that the darkness and cold, the frozen spiritual misery of recent times are breaking, cracking, and beginning to move, yielding to efforts to overcome spiritual muteness and moral paralysis. In this way, it is hoped, the immediacy of pain and sorrow, the primacy of tragedy and suffering in human life, may be transmuted into a spiritual and moral triumph. For the uniqueness of man lies in his capacity for self-transcendence.

RELIGIOUS PERSPECTIVES is therefore an effort to explore the *meaning* of God, an exploration which constitutes an aspect of man's intrinsic nature, part of his ontological substance. This Series grows out of an abiding concern that in spite of the release of man's creative energy which science has in part accomplished, this very science has overturned the essential order of nature. Shrewd as man's calculations have become concerning his means, his choice of ends which was formerly correlated with belief in God, with absolute criteria of conduct, has become witless. God is not to be treated as an exception to metaphysical principles, invoked to prevent their collapse. He is rather their chief exemplification, the sources of all potentiality. The personal reality of freedom and providence, of will and conscience, may demonstrate that "he who knows" commands a depth of consciousness inaccessible to the profane man, and is capable of that transfiguration which prevents the twisting of all good to ignominy. This religious content of experience is not within the province of science to bestow; it corrects the error of treating the scientific account as if it were itself metaphysical or religious; it challenges the tendency to make a religion of science—or a science of religion—a dogmatic act which destroys the moral dynamic of man. Indeed, many men of science are confronted with unexpected implications of their own thought and are beginning to accept, for instance, the trans-spatial and trans-temporal dimension in the nature of reality.

RELIGIOUS PERSPECTIVES attempts to show the fallacy of the

apparent irrelevance of God in history. This Series submits that
no convincing image of man can arise, in spite of the many ways
in which human thought has tried to reach it, without a philosophy of human nature and human freedom which does not ex-
clude God. This image of *Homo cum Deo* implies the highest
conceivable freedom, the freedom to step into the very fabric of
the universe, a new formula for man's collaboration with the
creative process and the only one which is able to protect man
from the terror of existence. This image implies further that the
mind and conscience are capable of making genuine discrimina-
tions and thereby may reconcile the serious tensions between the
secular and religious, the profane and sacred. The idea of the
sacred lies in what it *is,* timeless existence. By emphasizing timeless existence against reason as a reality, we are liberated in our
communion with the eternal, from the otherwise unbreakable
rule of "before and after." Then we are able to admit that all
forms, all symbols in religions, by their negation of error and
their affirmation of the actuality of truth, make it possible to experience that *knowing* which is above knowledge, and that
dynamic passage of the universe to unending unity.

God is here interpreted not as a heteronomous being issuing
commandments but as the *Tatt-Twam-Asi:* "Do unto others as
you would have others do unto you. For I am the Lord." This
does not mean a commandment from on high but rather a self-
realization through "the other"; since the isolated individual is
unthinkable and meaningless. Man becomes man by recognizing
his true nature as a creature capable of will and decision. For
then the divine and the sacred become manifest. And though he
believes in choices, he is no Utopian expecting the "coming of
the kingdom." Man, individually and collectively, is losing the
chains which have bound him to the inexorable demands of
nature. The constraints are diminishing and an infinity of choices
becomes available to him. Thus man himself, from the sources
of his ontological being, at last must decide what is the *bonum et
malum.* And though the anonymous forces which in the past

have set the constraints do indeed threaten him with total anarchy and with perhaps a worse tyranny than he experienced in past history, he nevertheless begins to see that preceding the moral issue is the cognitive problem: the perception of those conditions for life which permit mankind to fulfill itself and to accept the truth that beyond scientific, discursive knowledge is nondiscursive, intuitive awareness. And, I suggest, this is not to secularize God but rather to gather him into the heart of the nature of matter and indeed of life itself.

The volumes in this Series seek to challenge the crisis which separates, to make reasonable a religion that binds, and to present the numinous reality within the experience of man. Insofar as the Series succeeds in this quest, it will direct mankind toward a reality that is eternal and away from a preoccupation with that which is illusory and ephemeral.

For man is now confronted with his burden and his greatness: "He calleth to me, Watchman, what of the night? Watchman, what of the night?"[2] Perhaps the anguish in the human soul may be assuaged by the answer, by the *assimilation* of the person in God: "The morning cometh, and also the night: if ye will inquire, inquire ye: return, come."[3]

RUTH NANDA ANSHEN

[2] Isaiah 21:11.
[3] Isaiah 21:12.

1

The Aim of Yoga

The great interest evinced in Yoga and other occult doctrines by a large number of people, both in the East and in the West, is a clear indication of a growing thirst in men to know more about themselves, their birth and death, the real nature of the conscious principle animating them, and about the mystery surrounding the universe. There is nothing new in the expression of this impulse. It has been present in various forms from the day man began to lead the life of a rational being, from the day he began to use stone implements, of the crudest type, and to live a family and social life of the most primitive kind. That the thirst has always been present in one form or another is corroborated by the earliest relics of primitive men found in different parts of the earth. Undoubtedly there is a difference in the intensity of its expression and the form of its manifestation, but that the thirst has not abated is clear beyond the least shadow of doubt.

There appears to be a misconception in the minds of some people that Yoga offers an easy and convenient method for gaining access to the occult. This notion is especially prevalent in the West, and the idea persists that there are secret practices which can work wonders in leading men to the realm of the spirit. Such a conception is not peculiar to this era alone, but, in various forms, has been present from the remote past, ever since primitive man began to experiment with different methods to gain psychic powers, to invoke spirits and ghosts, to practice the art of magical healing, or to trade in sorcery and witchcraft. The men who practiced or professed these arts were always a source of wonder and attraction to novices desirous of attaining similar powers. The idea underlying this belief, which persists to this day, suggests that there are latent possibilities in the human mind which, when developed through appropriate methods, can place at the command of an adapt unseen, intelligent forces of nature which enable him to perform extraordinary feats utterly beyond the capacity of normal men. How far this concept is based on reality and how far it is a myth is the aim of this work to expound.

Properly speaking, Yoga is an adjunct to religion and has always been treated as such in India, the country of its birth. The word *Yoga* is derived from the Sanskrit root *yuj*, which means to yoke or join. As such, Yoga signifies the union of the individual soul with universal Consciousness or, in the language of the Upanishads, with the uncreated, all-pervading Brahman. In other words, the spiritual practices, classified under the general name Yoga, constitute different methods for the attainment of spiritual objectives, for verifying the doctrines formulated by prophets and sages, and for experiencing the Transcendent. Yoga is not something different or divorced from religion. It is the experimental part of it, offering ways and means to the properly qualified aspirants, prepared to undergo the discipline and to follow the methods suggested, to prove for themselves the validity of religious doctrines and the results attained by those who successfully pursued the path prescribed.

Yoga, as the empirical part of religion, is especially valuable in this age of reason as the growing intellect of the race demands some proof for the existence of the Transcendent Reality within the universe. Unless and until this proof is forthcoming, even in a subjective form, it will be increasingly difficult to reconcile the intellect with the existing dogmas of religion and agnosticism will continue to take a heavy toll from the ranks of scholars and men of science. From earliest times Yoga has provided the answer to the agnostic and the atheist in India. To the question, Can you prove the existence of a reality within the world of phenomena? the answer has been Yes. How? The answer, practice Yoga and see for yourself. It should not be supposed that India has not had its share of highly intelligent and vociferous skeptics and atheists. They existed even before the birth of Buddha in the sixth century before Christ, and under various guises have continued to spread their subversive doctrines to this day. Nevertheless, it is true that in spite of their opposition, Yoga continued to thrive and to be the chief instrument of realization for almost all the innumerable and, sometimes, mutually contending creeds and sects in India, thereby providing strong evidence of its vitality as well as its efficacy and popularity even under difficult conditions.

The validity of Yoga in its various forms as a tested method for gaining spiritual experience has never been doubted. On the other hand, the doctrine has remained surrounded by a halo that has continued undiminished to this day. Such a halo and such veneration, as Yoga now commands even in India, could never have been possible if from time to time its roots had not been watered by men of outstanding genius who brilliantly proved for themselves and others the possibility of the supreme achievement claimed for it. Because there exists a galaxy of extraordinary spiritual luminaries behind it, Yoga has been able to survive the onslaught of centuries and continues to this day to excite the curiosity and command the admiration of legions who accept it. There is ample evidence to show that the various methods used in Yoga were in vogue in India even in the Vedic age, long before the birth of Patanjali, the renowned author of Yoga-Sutras. To this great savant of the past, however, goes the credit for gathering the scattered threads of this hoary cult and formulating it, for the first time, into a methodological system of scientific experimentation and philosophy.

Divested of the superstition and myth that surround all religions, Yoga contains absolutely nothing that can be abhorrent to any faith or creed. On the other hand, it uses most of the methods advocated by the founders of great religions, mystics, and sages as a means to God-consciousness and to render the body a fit vehicle for spiritual illumination. Despite popular belief to the contrary, Yoga has never been considered to be a shortcut to self-realization. Although some writers on Yoga, even in the past, have claimed extraordinary efficacy for their particular method, the fact remains that this ancient system has never been considered as a means of easy approach to the Divine. On the contrary, all those who diligently pursued it did so with full realization that they were taking up a most serious quest and that they would be fortunate indeed if they attained some measure of success in it in their lifetime.

How seriously the quest is taken in India is, to some extent, evidenced by the large number of men who leave their homes and families to live in seclusion or in the company of masters to follow this path. Their number runs into millions. Apart from them, millions of men in different walks of life in India make Yoga an integral part of their lives, devoting to it all the time and energy they can spare, and even neglecting their worldly ambitions to achieve success in this enterprise. The life of most of these men is one great sacrifice to this holy quest. They have no delusions about the fact that they have entered upon an arduous undertaking, and have to submit completely to all the disciplines enjoined. They know that the prerequisites for an earnest study and practice of this venerable system are a recognition of this important fact, a readiness to make the sacrifice; and last, but not the least, to make it a permanent, integral part of one's life. The present sundry misconceptions about Yoga, treating it as a treasure house of easy-to-follow secret methods to experience the vision, Reality, or the psychic powers are entirely unfounded and often end in a painful harvest of disillusionment and frustration.

Many of the disciplines and practices of Yoga are common to

all great religions of mankind or, at least, to their esoteric aspects. The main difference is that in Yoga they have been brought into a methodological system divested of other ritual. This gives to Yoga the semblance of an independent cult. The word *yoga* is met for the first time in Vedas in the Katha Upanishad and some description of it is contained in Svetasvatra, the last of the early Upanishads. It is more frequently met with in Puranas, the epics and other later literature, and is sometimes synonymously used for *tapa* and *dhyana* (i.e., religious austerity and meditation). Basically Yoga is nothing more or less than systematized concentration. Fixity of attention, whether on a God or a goddess, on a symbol or a diagram, on the void or any material object, or whether on a *mantra* or any particular region of the body, is the main exercise of every ancient form of Yoga. It is at the same time the invariably met cornerstone of every religious discipline and occult practice known to man. Why it is so shall be explained at other places in this volume.

In one form or another Yoga, mental discipline and physical exercises combined, has been in vogue in different parts of the earth from time immemorial, forming a part—sometimes a repellent part—of primitive cults and creeds. Some of the unsavory practices continue to this day, incorporated into obscene rituals and ceremonies of some Yoga cults. In the light of these facts it is a mistake to treat Yoga as an independent system of exercises devised exclusively to bestow peace of mind or access to the occult world on those who practice it. But rather, it should be taken as a valuable system of tried religious practices, collected and coordinated, designed to form a much-needed adjunct to any religion of mankind for lending corroboration to the possibility of spiritual experience.

The modern tendency to divide Yoga into several different distinct and separate types, such as Karma-Yoga, Jnana-Yoga, Dhyana-Yoga, Mantra-Yoga, and the like, is based on an incorrect appraisal of the circumstances that led to the development of this science and an incorrect knowledge of its history. In the earliest religious literature of India no such distinction is made. It is true there must have always existed numerous schools of spiritual culture to cater to the needs of men of different tastes, different religious beliefs, different intellectual levels, and at different stages of moral development; and these schools, as is natural and as happens even now, must have designated their systems differently to invest them with importance and to attract disciples. But that difference extended only to the pattern of methods used and not to the fundamental concept of Yoga.

In the Bhagavad-Gita the enumeration of several forms of Yoga is an attempt at synthesis and every form has been praised. This is also clear from the reference made to the identity of *sankhya* and Yoga. In the Gita, from first to last, Yoga is treated as a powerful means toward emancipation, as an integral and essential part of man's religious zeal. The same view is taken in other well-known religious books of the Hindus. In the course of time the various methods of Yoga were also incorporated into the sacred books of Buddhists and penetrated to Tibet, China, Japan, and other places in the Far East. The diverse forms of Yoga, in vogue in India from very early times, embrace nearly all the methods adopted by people in different epochs and of different climes from the crude, primitive attempts made to gain supernatural power of healing, exorcism, black magic, prophecy, and the like to the subsequent supreme endeavor of spiritual illumination. Broadly defined the term *Yoga* can be applied to any systematic effort made by man to effect the assuagement of spiritual thirst by the use of suitable psychosomatic exercises out of the vast inventory of methods mentioned in Yoga texts and other religious documents. The main thing to be kept in mind is that Yoga is not an accidently discovered royal road to spiritual experience nor the secret treasure house of some magically effective methods for gaining uncanny psychical powers. In its diverse forms it is in reality the conglomeration of almost all the methods for the attainment of supernormal states of consciousness devised by the religious zeal of man. In other words, Yoga, in the real sense of the term and in the light of the purpose for which it is employed, is to the supersensory or spiritual part of man what empirical science is to his visible or physical part.

Yoga provides methods for the attestation of spiritual truths, but the laboratory is the man himself. In this sublime enterprise he has to experiment upon himself to know the real facts about his own existence, or about the entity who never reveals his own nature to him from birth to the last day of his pilgrimage on earth, and keeps him perpetually mystified about his past and future, a prey to doubts and misgivings from the day he begins to think coherently to the end. It never was and never can be a readily available talisman to bridge the yawning gulf between the seen and the unseen, between the physical and the super-physical for all and sundry who undertake it. On the other hand, the mental and physical constitution of the seeker and the diligence and purity of purpose with which he devotes himself to the effort are of paramount importance in determining the measure of success he achieves. It must be clearly understood that Yoga does not provide, as is sometimes supposed, a way of escape from the earthly part of our lives or a back-door entrance to the Divine for the evasion of religious obligations and spiritual responsibilities—speaking in universal, not parochial, terms—that devolve on man.

Patanjali, in his Yoga-Sutras, introducing the doctrine for the first time as a distinct and methodical system of spiritual exercises and philosophy, defines Yoga as restraint of the fluctuations of mind-stuff. In other words, it means a condition of mental arrest in which the superphysical existence of consciousness, beyond the range of the senses and the mind, becomes perceptible to the initiate. According to Yoga-Sutras one of the attributes necessary in the aspirant is Astikta, or belief in God. This belief is not to be taken in any restricted sense. In order to be qualified as an "Astikta," one may believe in an anthropomorphic God or a multitude of gods or a God without form, or a Transcendent Reality in the shape of Brahman or Shiva or Divinity in any conceivable mold, but he must believe in Vedas and in the spiritual destiny of man. The followers of *sankhya,* which does not advocate a belief in God, but in the plurality of individual souls and *prakrati,* or matter, exploit Yoga for the verification of their own tenets. Similarly Buddhists use it for establishing the validity of their own conceptions that human existence is a series of incarnations not of an individual soul, but of a combination of elements, until after righteous endeavor it terminates in *nirvana* or cessation from the cycle of births and deaths.

The monotheists, the dualists, and the pantheists in India look up to and use Yoga for the demonstration of their particular spiritual beliefs and dogmas. The Vedantists practice it to prove that the soul or *Atman* and Brahman are one and the phenomenal world is an illusion born of the action of *maya,* an unfathomable and inexplicable conditioning factor, which envelops the *Atman* in a veil of myth. The Saivites practice their own forms of Yoga to prove that the universe is the manifestation of *shakti,* the creative and active aspect of the Shiva-Shakti combination, the two-in-one attribute of Para Shiva, the lord of creation, who is both the creator and the created, by combining the conscious principle and the conscious creative energy in one. In fact, all sects, creeds, and faiths in India, and there are many of them, depend on Yoga for the demonstration of their truths and the verification of their varied and, sometimes, diametrically opposed beliefs.

It is therefore obvious that Yoga has to be viewed from a broader angle than is sometimes used at present. Even in recent years the results attained through the practice of Yoga have been variously evaluated and described by the religious luminaries of India. The Vedantists, the Buddhists, the worshipers of *Shakti,* or Shakts, the Vaisnavites and all the rest, who claim success in Yoga, describe their experience in terms of the doctrines and beliefs of their own creed. This means that the final state of Yoga, namely, the ultimate condition of mental arrest or Samādhi, is not always the same but varies with the individual and the faith he owns. From this it follows clearly that those who wish to take up the practice of Yoga, with a definite understanding that it would lead to such-and-such a condition, and those who foster this belief among the people not well versed in the history and the entire application of the system, are not treading on solid ground.

This misconception not only leads to wrong endeavor, disappointment, and frustration but also to a tremendous waste of human energy. The only reasonable and safe attitude would be to treat Yoga as a systematized form of religious striving, needing lifelong attention and sacrifice, for a successful consummation, as has always been recognized; but what that consummation would be no one can be sure from the start. If the exercises and the disciplines enjoined are followed scrupulously one may expect a measure of success, provided the body and the mind are already in a certain state of maturity, but what form that success would take, what would be the nature of the ecstasy, what mental phenomena would be witnessed and what shape the vision would take, no one can predict. It is thus evident that the stereotyped goal of an unfluctuating and unmodified state of consciousness mentioned by Patanjali does not hold true for all. In the Yoga-Sutras he postulates the existence of Iswara, not as the Almighty Creator of the Universe and the ultimate source and refuge of all that exists, but as a sort of superior overself that helps earnest seekers to gain *mokṣa,* or liberation, with the practice of Yoga. This concept of the ultimate is at variance with the Brahman of Vedanta, the Shiva of Saivite, and Vishnu of the Vaisnavite cults in India. Such a variation in the concept of the Transcendent Reality, depending on the pattern of the vision experienced in *samadhi,* provides an irrefutable testimony to the fact that the supersensory experience of even the highest adapts in Yoga in the past has not been identical, but unmistakably varied even in respect to the fundamental truths.

The main problem, on which no light has been thrown by any writer, ancient or modern, is: How does the extraordinary condition of consciousness associated with Yoga and other forms of spiritual effort come about? How does the practitioner find himself wafted, in the state of trance or Samādhi to regions of omnipotence, transcending the narrow human limits, or to regions of deathlessness, glory, and incomparable bliss? Although the ecstasy of a modern mystic or Yogi denotes a tremendous leap forward from the self-induced trance of a Shaman, the experience of a state of power with vastly extended knowledge or of a direct contact with higher beings or higher states of consciousness, which is common to both, reveals an undeniable similarity in the basic characteristics of the two. In dealing with Yoga we are, therefore, faced by a historical problem, stretching across vast spans of time, that has its roots in the uncanny performances of the medicine-man and the witchdoctor in primitive societies and its branches in the varied experience of Western mystics: the Sufis of the Middle East, the Taoists of China, the Zen masters of Japan, the Yogis of India and Tibet in more recent historic times.

On account of the fact that there is a radical difference in the concept of Yoga, as presented in this volume, with corroboration from ancient canonical texts and standard books on the subject, and the generally accepted ideas, current today, it is necessary to make this distinction clear at the outset in order to avoid confusion. According to my view all systems of Yoga embody divergent methods for the metamorphosis of consciousness. The real aim of Yoga is not to cause an obstruction in the normal flow of thought by sustained efforts of concentration, but to open new areas of perception in the brain capable of manifesting a trans-human state of consciousness. The ideas expressed by some modern writers that the practice of concentration, carried to the required degree, can enable the Sadhaka to keep out both the sensory impressions, coming from outside, and the subconscious impulses, invading the mind from within, and in this state of freedom to experience the transcendent, do not at all present a correct picture of the processes released by Yoga or of the ultimate state to which it leads. There is no agreement at the present moment between the principles underlying Yoga and the concepts of modern psychology and, therefore, any attempt to explain one in terms of the other cannot lead to an understanding of the causes that generate the supernormal states of consciousness associated with Yoga.

The aim of Yoga is to accelerate a natural process, already at work in the human organism: to mold the brain to a higher state of awareness. Modern psychology has no inkling of this process and, therefore, does not take it seriously into account in its treatment of the mind and its problems. There is no recognition among present-day psychologists of the obvious fact that the human brain is still evolving toward a yet unknown destination. This being the case, psychology can as yet have no jurisdiction over the province covered by Yoga. It is for this reason that, in spite of its antiquity and the overwhelming testimony of hundreds of top-rank intellects of India, the validity of Yoga as a means to gain transcendent states of consciousness still remains to be accepted by the scholars of today, and the whole subject is obscure and controversial. Even in India there is a great divergence of opinion concerning the efficacy of the various practices as well as about the ultimate condition toward which Yoga leads. Thus for Sankara, the exercise of the intellect to discriminate between the real and the unreal, before the actual beginning of the various steps of Yoga, is necessary in order to reach the supreme state; while in the Yoga-Sutras of Patanjali no such condition is imposed. In Gita, the greatest stress is laid on passionate love and longing for the Deity whether manifesting itself in a form or in formlessness; Ramanuja, another famous exponent of Vedanta, believes in acts of daily worship, devout meditation (*upasana*), and self-surrender as the surest way of reaching Brahman. He says in Sri Bhasya (iii.2.23): "It is only in the state of perfect endearment, i.e., in meditation bearing the character of deep devotion, that intuitive knowledge of Brahman is gained and not in any other state."

The Vedas lay stress on the performance of daily observances, austerity and *dhyana* (meditation), and the earlier Upanishads

on righteous conduct, control of the senses and meditation on
Brahman as the means to liberation. The Upanishads, which
show an advance over the ritualistic practices (*karma-kanda*) of
the Vedas as a result of social and mental evolution achieved
during the course of centuries intervening between the two, assign
a higher place to intellectual discrimination in the pursuit of
mokṣa (liberation) than to religious rites and daily Karma (agni-
hotra, etc.). Thus it is said in the Mundaka-Upanishad (iii.1.8):
"It, i.e., the Brahman, is not comprehended through the eye, nor
through speech, nor through the other senses, nor is it attained
through austerity or Karma (daily performance of religious
duties). When one becomes purified in mind with the blessings
of a rightly discriminating intellect then only can one realize that
indivisible Self through meditation." According to Bhagavad-
Purana utter surrender to the Lord paves the way to emancipation. "Those who dedicate every day," it says, 10.26.15, "their
passion, anger, fear, love, unity and friendship to Hari, attain
Him." This is confirmed in Bhagavad-Gita (ix.34) in the words of
Sri Krishna addressed to Arjuna: "Fix your mind on Me, be devoted to Me, make obeisance to Me, worship Me, thus uniting
yourself to Me and entirely depending on Me you shall come to
Me." Krishna repeats this promise again more emphatically at the
end of the discourse (xviii.66) thus: "Surrendering all duties
(*dharmas*) come to Me alone for refuge"; "Grieve not, I shall
absolve thee of all sins."

The greatest emphasis among all the factors conducive to liberation has been laid on detachment, intense devotion, and purity
of mind by most of the spiritual luminaries of India. The possibility of emancipation for one who has not purified himself is
categorically denied in the Katha Upanishad (1.11.24). "One who
has not desisted from evil conduct, who has not his senses under
control, whose mind is not concentrated and free from anxiety
cannot attain this Self through knowledge." The preliminary
practices of Yoga are, in actual fact, meant for effecting the much-
needed purification of the bodily organs, the nervous system and

the mind. Without this purification the practice of concentration, *dharma* and *dhyana* becomes fruitless. For this reason some of the renowned Yoga saints in India consider the dry disciplines of Yoga an impediment rather than an aid to realization as compared to purity of mind and intense longing for the Supreme. Surdas in his Brahmragita ridicules the idea of Yoga without *bhakti* (devotion) serving as a means for the attainment of God. In his Sursagar he makes the following observation: "In whose company am I to talk. He talks of Yoga in which all taste of life is burnt up."

Kabir, another famous Yoga saint, presents the same idea in these words: "Without devotion to God the wicked go astray. Whomever I approach for my deliverance is himself caught in the net. Yogis say Yoga is best and there is nothing else. Hairy and shaven Sadhus (ascetics) claim that they have found *siddhi* (psychic powers, perfection). The Pandit, the warrior, the poet, the patron—each says he alone is great. . . . Leave passion to your right and left and hold on to the feet of Hari (the Lord)." Sankaradeva, the far-famed saint of Assam who flourished in the fifteenth century, conveys the same idea when he says: "Thou hast muttered spells (*mantras*), undergone austerities. . . . Yoga and logic have been mastered by thee, yet clouded is thy mind, for without devotion there can be no salvation. All piety resideth in the name of Rama; this is the essential message of all holy books." The earnest attitude of utter surrender and overwhelming devotion is beautifully expressed in the Mahanarayan Upanishad (38.1) in these words: "May the Supreme accept me. May the Blissful accept me. May the Supreme alone that is Blissful accept me. O Lord, being one among Thy creatures, I am Thy child. End the dreary dream of the sorrowful existence that I experience. For that I offer myself as an oblation unto Thee, O Lord, together with the *prana* [life energy] Thou hast infused in me."

The whole spiritual literature of India is pervaded through and through with the utterances of venerated sages and seers, from the age of the Upanishads to the present day, proclaiming purity of mind, detachment from the fret and fever of the world, extreme devotion to and constant meditation on the Deity as the most effective means to self-realization. The regimented system of Yoga, as propounded by Patanjali, beginning with *yama* and ending in Samādhi, is not earlier than the beginning of the Christian era, though the practices enumerated must have been in use from time immemorial. In the Vedas and the Upanishads *tapas* (austerity), *mitya karma* (daily observances), *dhyana* (meditation), bhakti (devotion), *vairagya* (detachment), *viveka* (discrimination), *brahmẹarya* (continence), *upasana* (constant, devout and reverent thought), *jnana* (intuitive knowledge), and the like are all said to be the channels through which one can attain knowledge of the Reality. As Yoga etymologically denotes union or, in other words, the merger of the embodied individual soul with the all-pervading Isvara or Brahman, it follows that every practice or method, whether adopted singly or in combination with others, which tends to bring about this fusion can be called Yoga. For this reason Bhagavad Gita, Puranas, and other books mention various forms of Yoga: Dhyana-Yoga, Karma-Yoga, Jnana-Yoga, Mantra-Yoga, Laya-Yoga, Bhakti-Yoga, Hatha-Yoga, Surta-Sabda-Yoga, etc. The system adumbrated by Patanjali is sometimes called Raja-Yoga in contradistinction to Mantra-Yoga and Hatha-Yoga of the Tantras. Several of the methods used in one form of Yoga are more or less common to other forms also, with more emphasis on this or that practice than on others.

Since every form of Yoga is designed to lead to *mokṣa* (liberation) on attainment of knowledge of the self it follows that *çitta-vrtti nirodhah* (restraint of the fluctuations of the mind-stuff) is not the only way to attain the unitive state but that it can be obtained, perhaps more easily and with greater fulfillment, through other paths, such as the path of *bhakti* (devotion), *jnana* (intuitive knowledge), *karma* (religious observances with selfless action), and *upasana* (constant devout thought of the Deity) also. Purity of mind, detachment, self-discipline, and chastity are the common ingredients necessary to be acquired on any of these paths. That the goal of all forms of Yoga is the same is asserted by the Gita (xiii.24 and 25) in these words: "Some by meditation behold the Self in themselves with the help of pure reason, others by proceeding along the path of knowledge and others, again, by treading the path of action. Others, however, not knowing this, take to worship (*upasana*) by hearing from others, and they, too, who are thus intent on hearing, transcend death." From this it is clear that all forms of Yoga ultimately lead to a state of inner illumination. This point is further clarified in the Gita (V.5), while discussing the relative merits of Sankhya and Yoga schools of self-discipline: "The supreme state which is attained by Sankhya is also reached by Yoga. He who sees that Sankhya and Yoga are one really sees."

The implication of the synthesis, attempted in Bhagavad-Gita, is obvious. To the casual observer it merely signifies that all paths ultimately lead to God. For the common man the same view is also expressed in Gita (iv.II): "By whatsoever path men approach Me even so do I meet them, for all men follow My path from all sides." For an earnest seeker, however, who wishes to go to the root of the matter, this position gives rise to a host of problems which must be answered if Yoga is to be made acceptable to the modern highly sophisticated intellect. If constant practice of meditation in a fixed posture with regulated breathing (*pranayama*) and eyes fixed on the tip of the nose or the place between the eyebrows, can lead to the same supersensory state, after years of hard endeavor, to which mere repetition of the name of the Lord or the *mantra "Om"* without a regular posture or *pranayama,* or mere singing the praises of God in a devotional frame of mind, or pure intellectual deliberation on the Real and the Unreal, or simple performance of daily work in a spirit of dedication, or any other act of worship can pave the way, it undeniably signifies that the conventional techniques of Yoga are not the only means to gain access to higher states of consciousness or to the occult areas of the mind. On the other hand, it shows that there are varying states and varying degrees of responsiveness in the minds of the seekers. This accounts for the diverse nature of the methods, some easy and some difficult, that must be adopted, according to the aptitude and the state of development of each seeker, in order to lead to a successful conclusion of the endeavor.

The modern books on Yoga, presenting a stereotyped version of the Yoga-Sutras of Patanjali or of Hatha-Yoga, as propounded in the ancient manuals on the subject, have been instrumental in creating a wrong impression, especially in the West, that the practices enjoined in these systems induce a special psycho-mental condition, by the elimination of sensory impressions and thought, in which the spirit, liberated from these fetters, perceives its own glorious, ever blissful and immortal nature. If it is accepted that a transcendent state of consciousness can proceed only from the suppression of the activity of the mind, and by completely shutting out stimuli coming from the senses, the question immediately arises as to how, in that case, does the same state of transcendence supervene in the case of a Bakhta (devotee) or a Karma-Yogi (man of selfless action), who merely adores the Lord in his heart or surrenders all his actions to Him? In such cases as well as in that of the illuminati who possess the condition from birth, the higher state of consciousness can manifest itself, and has indeed manifested itself on occasions, without the arduous mental training and rigid disciplines of regimented Yoga. This is an enigma hard to explain in the light of the current psychological explanations offered for the final state of Samadhi attained by Yoga. However difficult it may be to solve the riddle, the fact remains that in all authoritative canonical books and other spiritual literature of the Hindus the equality of opportunity for the attainment of the highest state to all the aspirants, namely, the orthodox Yogi, the man of dedicated action, the devotee, the discriminating intellectual and the man of unwavering faith and piety, has been unreservedly guaranteed.

This possibility is recognized clearly by Patanjali in Sutra I of the fourth book of his Yoga-Sutras wherein he says: "*Siddhis* (psychic powers and perfection) proceed from birth or from drugs

or from spells (*mantras*) or from austerity or *samadhi*." This
aphorism plainly signifies that the *siddhis* resulting from concentration and *samadhi*, gained through the methods advocated
by him, are naturally present in some men at birth or can be
attained by the use of certain drugs or by spells or austerity
(*tapas*). In this way Patanjali has equated the possession of
psychic powers and mystical faculties, exhibited by some individuals as a natural endowment at birth, and the trancelike
states, caused by certain drugs or by the casting of spells or by
fasting and other forms of austerity, with the *Siddhis* proceeding
from *samadhi* and the long, elaborate course of self-discipline and
concentration prescribed by him. Critically examined this passage
is of tremendous significance. If drugs and spells can bestow the
same intuitive state of knowledge and the same psychic gifts as
result from the extremely arduous discipline of Yoga, leading to
cessation of *karma* and to liberation, the ultimate goal of all
yogic disciplines, it means that potions and charms can be as
effective in cutting asunder the veil of *maya* and the fetters of
karma as all the virtues demanded and the difficult efforts required in the practice of Yoga for many years—self-sacrifice,
devotion, and righteousness—all dedicated to God.

Such an idea would, no doubt, strike those who believe in the
infallibility of divine justice as most revolting. It would equate
the mescaline addict, sunk in sensuality, with the mystic and the
saint whose immaculate life has been one long sacrifice to a holy
cause. Obviously there is a veil of mystery surrounding the entire
subject. This prevents us from probing more deeply into the
inner recesses of the spirit in order to reconcile the striking
anomalies which bewilder those who would like to have a rational
explanation for the varied phenomena attending spiritual unfoldment, in order to obliterate their doubts. All the issues and
anomalies, mentioned above, will be discussed at their proper
places in other chapters of this volume. It is here sufficient to
point them out in order to show that Yoga, in the proper sense
of the term, embraces a wide variety of methods and practices

prescribed to gain a supernormal state of consciousness that has been an invariable adornment of the enlightened sages, prophets, and mystics of the past. Many of them never practiced Yoga in their life and were born with the faculty already developed in the womb. Others gained it through frequenting the company of holy men and hearing the descriptions of the supreme state from their lips, others by prayer, still others by austerity and self-mortification; some by practicing the disciplines of Yoga for an incredibly short spell of time and some by sudden insight, a sudden flash of intuitive knowledge, which, like a streak of lightning, clears the darkness of the mind (*avidya*), leaving them amazed and breathless, blessed with a freshly gained, glorious vision that penetrated into the nature of things.

By diverse paths and in diverse forms the seers of India, the Taoists of China, the Buddhist arhats, the Sufis of the Middle East, the Zen masters in Japan, the Siddhas of Tibet and the mystics of the West attained through Yoga the fusion of the individual with universal consciousness, interpreting their experience in diverse ways. In some cases the fusion might have been momentary, in others of longer duration, lasting for hours, and in still others existing permanently. But that the impact of each experience was most overpowering, is clear beyond a doubt. The complexity of the phenomenon, its varied nature, and the fact that one, witnessing it in himself, is completely carried away for the time being by the overwhelming nature of the experience have always stood in the way of an intelligent understanding and consistent expression of the condition. Hardly any one of them could coherently express what he had apprehended. No one of them was the same after the experience as he had been before it. No one of them fell below the stature he attained as a result of it.

The very first contact with the Divine, the very first taste of the indescribable experience, the very first sight of the Ineffable changed the lives and metamorphosed the inner being of those who succeeded in attaining the Transcendent. They then pined day and night for the same experience and were infinitely more happy in the inner than in the outer world. It does not materially affect the transformed condition achieved if there are great divergences in their accounts of the supreme experience. It also does not matter if there are wide differences in the experience itself. The fact that one of them was blessed with the vision of an adored Savior, another with that of a venerated Prophet, another with the glorious image of a preconceived God, or another with the vision of a formless but all-pervading and almighty Conscious Being, does not falsify the experience, but only accentuates the varied nature of the phenomenon and the inadequacy of any current explanation offered for it. What matters is that the basic characteristics of the mystical trance or *samadhi* are present in varying forms in the experience: an overmastering sense of wonder at the extraordinary occurrence, the unutterably glorious nature of the vision, a powerful feeling of awe combined with inexpressible happiness, overflow of love, and entrancement or a state of complete or partial oblivion to the world. Last, but not the least, there is the vivid consciousness of a higher existence or of submersion into an ocean of knowledge in which all that was obscured is now explained.

This is the aim of Yoga: the elevation of the narrow, fear-ridden and desire-tormented human consciousness to a state of indescribable beauty, glory, and bliss. This is the aim of all religious striving and spiritual endeavor, this transmutation of the human mind, culminating in its liberation from the chains of ego, insatiable desire, and fear of death. But this far-reaching transformation of personality is never achieved by one's efforts alone. The as yet inscrutable laws of heredity must have prepared the soil for the efforts to bear fruit. Then only can the mortal become immortal and the earthly divine. Then only does a fortunate seeker gain access to the indefinable inner world, the glorious realm of consciousness to which no human sense and no man-made device can penetrate: a world, infinitely vaster and infinitely more mysterious and breath-taking, than the material universe, which can only be approached directly by the knowing self, without the mediation of the senses and the intrusion of the intellect, for it is as far removed from the world, apprehended by the mind, and explored by the intellect as the brilliant light of the noonday sun is from the dark shadows of the night.

The well-known Christian mystic writing under the name of Dionysius toward the end of the fifth century has tried to portray this state in these words: "The super-unknown, the super-luminous and loftiest height, wherein the simple and absolute and unchangeable mysteries are cloaked in the superlucent darkness of hidden mystic silence, which supershines most brightly in the blackest night, and, in the altogether intangible and unseen, fills the eyeless understanding with superbeautiful brightness. . . . And thou, dear friend, in thy intent practice of mystical contemplation, leave behind both thy senses and thy intellectual operations, and all things known by sense and intellect, and all things which are not and which are, and set thyself, as far as may be, to unite thyself in *unknowing* with Him, who is above all things and knowledge, for by being purely free and absolute, out of self and all things, thou shalt be led up to the ray of the divine darkness, stripped from all and loosed from all."

Compare this with the description contained in the Mandukya Upanishad (i.7): "They consider the fourth, i.e., the Turiya state (the crowning state of Yoga) to be that which is not conscious of the internal world, nor conscious of the external world, nor conscious of both the worlds, nor a mass of consciousness, nor simple consciousness, nor unconsciousness; which is unseen, beyond empirical dealings, beyond the grasp (of the organs of action), uninferable, unthinkable, indescribable; whose valid proof consists in one single belief in the Self; in which all phenomena cease; and which is unchanging, auspicious and nondual. That is the Self, and that is to be known."

It is obvious that both these quotations refer to the same condition, to the same incommunicable, mystical experience, in which the overpowered intellect reels back defeated from the arena where the spirit unfolds itself. The crowning achievement of Yoga and every true and healthy form of spiritual striving can be the same. Only the psychological constitution of the individuals causes the variations.

2

How This Aim Is Achieved

The mystical state is still an incomprehensible phenomenon of consciousness. The range of its expression is so varied and the area of its manifestations so extensive that it is difficult at this stage of our knowledge to assign any well-marked limits to it. In its most common form the time of its occurrence and the duration of its operation are unpredictable. The flash of inner illumination may last only for a few moments, like the dazzling brightness of a meteor shooting across the sky in the darkness of night, or it may continue for an hour or several hours or even days at a time. It may occur once in a lifetime, or a few times in one's life, or daily, or every night at different hours. Sri Ramakrishna's ecstasies lasted for both short and long durations and, sometimes, entrancement occurred several times in a day. St. Angela of Foligno had her highest vision of God three times, and Plotinus, according to his disciple Porphyry, four times in a period of six years. In the case of a clergyman quoted by William James, "the soul opened into the infinite . . . with ineffable joy and exultation" only once, while in the case of Margiad Evans the state of union was of long duration, extending even to sleep. Shams-i-Tabriz, the mystic poet of Persia, was perennially in a state of divine intoxication: "In a place even beyond outer space, in a tract without a trace of shadow, soul and body transcending, I live in the soul of my Loved One anew," he says.

The variation between one kind of experience and another, even in a few sample cases pertaining to different people and relating to different periods, is so great and so unaccountable that it is extremely difficult to understand that they are allied to one another. The number of those belonging to the regular order of ecstatics is comparatively limited. There are many people who at one time or another in their lives experience the beatific vision suddenly, in unexpected ways or under strange circumstances, and feel themselves in a new world or a new order of things. As if temporarily gifted with a new kind of perception, they see their surroundings transformed into a dreamland, a realm of inexpressible glory in which, forgetting for a while who they are, they taste the joy of a liberated existence, unencumbered by the problems and obsessions of the earth. Or the whole cosmic panorama may appear so changed, so magnified, so full of grandeur and sublimity that the mind reels under the impact.

The same experience in a more or less intense form occurs to many people in dreams or in the state between waking and dreaming. They see themselves as if in heavenly surroundings in a highly exalted and blissful state, drinking in the beauty and the glory of the paradise around them, or viewing a celestial object or a godlike being with a rapture that is unknown to the waking consciousness." The majority of people who have any type of mystical experience on rare occasions in their life are often reluctant to relate these intimate episodes of their being to others, under the mistaken idea that the occurrence might savor of the abnormal, or that such an experience, being extremely rare or peculiar to them alone, might be ridiculed by those to whom they narrate the incident. There are other variations also. The rapture, with an instantaneous break through the normal state of awareness into a superearthly plane of existence in which one is swallowed by a flood of inexpressible bliss, might be evoked by a strain of melody, a beautiful object, the atmosphere of a holy shrine, or even by the embrace of love. The power of expression and the sense of evaluation of their own feelings and mental states vary with different people. Some are prone to depict even trivial occurrences in a highly embellished and colorful language, while in the case of others a restricted power of expression stands in the way of an adequate presentation of remarkable experiences which can rank with those recorded of well-known mystics and saints.

Viewed from a rational aspect, experiences of a transcendent nature, occurring in persons who never practised Yoga or any other form of spiritual discipline, nor were particularly devotional or even deeply religious in the ordinary sense of the term, present a riddle which is not explicable on the basis of any of the numerous solutions proposed for the problem. No one can deny the basic similarity between the ecstatic states described by Wordsworth, Tennyson, Charlotte Bronte, C. E. Montague, Plato, Whitman, Marcel Proust, Nietzsche, and a host of other writers, thinkers, and those recorded by reputed mystics of the West and renowned yogis of the East. There must be countless other intelligent men and women of many countries and cultures who had this experience at one time or another like a bolt from the blue, during the course of an ordinary, strictly mundane life, and who had either no inclination or no literary ability to describe it in words. It appears unbelievable that lifelong devotion to the Deity and sacrifice of all the enticements and pleasures of earth, with ceaseless observance of the rigid disciplines of Yoga, should fail to elicit any reward or, here also in rare cases, should only be recompensed in almost the same way as some individuals, among the worldly mass of mankind, are rewarded without having made any effort whatsoever to deserve it. But it is a hard, historical reality which, so far, has not been satisfactorily explained.

The unitive state may range from a single, momentary sense of oneness with nature with a blissful release from the world-weary selfhood, felt in a sudden upsurge of a new, unidentified

life from within, to experience, described by the well-known
mystic Jacob Boehme when he "felt" in a flash of lightning that
the gate of his soul was opened and he saw and knew what no
books could "teach," to the state of perennial ecstasy, described
by Abhinava-Gupta in these words:

> O, Bhairava-Natha [Lord Shiva]
> Thou Refuge of the friendless, Supreme Being,
> Pervading both the sentient and the insentient worlds,
> Pure Consciousness, One, Eternal, Infinite . . .
> By the potency of Thy Grace the world today
> Appears to me to be Thy Person, O Mahestra,
> And Thee as my Atman ever more, and so I feel
> This whole creation as my very self. . . .

The taproot of mystical experience lies in consciousness, and
consciousness in different individuals is not the same. The one
great lesson which this experience brings home to us is that the
very fundamental constituent of personality, namely consciousness, varies in different people. When we say that a certain man
is intelligent and another dull or that one is more aesthetic or
sensitive than the other, we often invest him with a conscious
personality like our own, but with the difference that he is more
or less intelligent, or more or less sensitive. This is a mistake
based on a fundamentally erroneous way of thinking; for as no
two faces and no two streams of thought are exactly alike, so no
two units or pools of consciousness, representing the personality
or the outer area of manifestation of the soul, are alike in any
two persons, including even identical twins. Each unit of human
consciousness has, as it were, its own volume, its own area, its
own depth, its own power of perception, grasp, and penetration.
It has its own memory, scale of passion and intensity of desire.
Each personality has a distinct stamp, a peculiar pattern clearly
embossed on it, to which it conforms more or less throughout its
life. In the genuine mystical state this everyday personality that
has its roots in the deepest strata of the human mind evaporates
for a time, opening its otherwise strongly enclosed precincts to
the influx of a torrent that floods the now empty enclosure with

a new kind of life, a new pattern of consciousness, and, overflowing the former narrow boundaries, causes mixed feelings of wonderment, exaltation, bliss, awe, and a sense of all-pervasiveness, infinity, and sovereignty in the now eclipsed original personality, a thin shadow of which still lurks in the mind. If this shadow did not survive it would be impossible for the normal consciousness to have any recollection of the extraordinary experience. One would come back from it, like a man awakening from dreamless slumber, without the recollection of any impression received in that state. Even in *nirvikalpa samadhi* (contemplation) an attenuated shadow of the normal self continues to function and brings back the memory of the stupendous vision seen. Quivering and throbbing the overshadowed self, shrunken almost to a pinpoint before the immeasurable Presence that now encompasses it, has still the faculty left to make a comparison between itself and the veritable Universe of Being, unlike anything known to it on the earth, absolutely beyond description, with which for a breathless interval and with unutterable rapture it finds itself in complete identity, like a drop of water merged with the ocean to which it belongs.

The description of the Cosmic Being contained in the eleventh chapter of the Bhagavad-Gita shows overawed Arjuna (the human element still left even in the highest form of mystical contemplation) in a state of utter surrender, confronted by the infinite, indescribable Universe of Life, revealed to him in a divine vision through the grace of Krishna (the Cosmic Self). If mystical union is a genuine experience of the human mind, and not merely a delusive state, there must be a concordance in the essentials of the fully blossomed state experienced by the visionaries of all religions, irrespective of the period or the culture to which they belong. The surest way to cast a doubt on the validity of the phenomenon, and thereby on the fundamental basis of religion itself, is for the adherents of one faith to belittle or to question the genuineness of the experience described by the contemplatives of another religion or cult. The tendency among some writers on mysticism to devaluate the supreme experience, depicted in the Upanishads, of the absorption of Atman into the attributeless Brahman, in which one is lost to everything that can be apprehended by the intellect, reveals only a lack of firsthand knowledge of the crowning state of mystical contemplation. The view expressed by Dean Inge that the highest state of Indian mystics is that of inertness, of total self-loss and annihilation springs from a sectarian concept of the Divinity. To hold that the Supreme Being conforms to this or that image or can be experienced only in this or that form is to bring Him, who is beyond the furthest reach of our thought, down to the prosaic level of a puny human being. The view is self-contradictory, for were the experience of a nihilistic character, with total loss of the observing power of the soul, how could the seers bring back a vivid description of it, even in negative terms—that it is not this . . . ; not this . . . ; not this . . .—on returning to the normal state?

It is obvious that even among intellectuals there is a misconception about the real nature of the ecstatic state. For one who never had the experience it is impossible to imagine the condition of the contemplative's mind at the time of the flight of the soul toward the Ineffable. Were God or the Absolute to be apprehended as we apprehend the objects of senses or the abstract ideas present in our mind, it would reduce the whole phenomenon of mysticism to everyday occurrences of the material world, perhaps in a more grandiose, more impressive and more exalted form, but a mundane experience nevertheless. By no stretch of the imagination can a supersensory knowledge of the Godhead be likened to knowledge in the ordinary sense of the term. There must occur the development of a new faculty, the opening of a new channel of perception or a radical transformation and enhancement of the normal powers of observation of the soul to enable it to have even a fleeting glimpse of the Supreme Being. Since God, as He is conceived in all Semitic religions, is the Maker or Master of the human soul and according to Vedanta is the Absolute as also the Atman itself, it follows in either case that in order to apprehend Him the soul has to transcend the limitations of the flesh in the former case; or those, imposed on it by *maya,* in the latter; and to attain a transhuman state of knowledge where this infinite Ocean of Being or this boundless Conscious Substratum of the whole universe can be known.

This means, in other words, that the human soul in order to apprehend the infinite must cease to be finite itself and must partake for the time being of superhuman attributes and a superhuman state of cognition to have even a transient or fragmentary knowledge of Him or That, who is normally beyond the grasp of his sensory equipment and mind. In this state of transcendence, in this rapturous union between the Creator, the Master, or the Substance of the soul and the soul itself, in both the Eastern and Western senses of the phenomenon, how can the enthralled mystic, transported to other realms of existence, determine where his light of knowledge ends and the glory of God begins? Like a grain of salt dropped into an ocean, his narrow personality melts and spreads the moment it comes in contact with the shoreless stream of life, surrendering joyously all its mental possessions, shedding cheerfully every individual trait that stands between it and the rapturous, incorporeal oceanic state of Being, happy beyond measure to be one with the glorious, everlasting All instead of an isolated mortal tormented by desire, death, and decay. "Thou wert ever close to me," says the famous mystical poetess of Kashmir, Lalladed, "and yet I searched for Thee till the evening shadows fell. But, lo, when at last I saw Thee in myself, I at once realized my distinction from the earth, that is, the body and identity with Thee." At another place she adds: "Having known Thee, I find that Thou art all and I nothing." What some Western writers treat as "extinction" or "annihilation" after reading the description of "union with Brahman" or *nirvana* is, in actual fact, the effacement of the dividing line between the individual and the Cosmic Consciousness. Once transformed into an ocean, who would care to return to the uncertainty and the torment of a transient bubble?

The mistake is caused by the erroneous supposition that in

these high states of mystical union there is a complete obliteration of personality. This does not occur, since such an event would rob the supreme experience of all its happiness and grandeur. The same misunderstanding can result from the term *fana* used in Sufi literature. The word *fana* connotes extinction. The ego-bound, narrow human personality has to efface itself to make room for a higher state of Being to transcend the limitations, imposed by the senses, and to be in a position to grasp the hitherto Intangible and to know the previously Unknowable. When the contact takes place it has the effect of Divine Intoxication, so beautifully expressed by the Sufi poets. In this state of *sat-chit-ananda* (existence, consciousness, bliss) the enraptured soul breaking the restraining bonds of the ego loses all idea of the body, the world, and the objects of the senses in the contemplation of a surpassingly blissful, intensely alive, and extremely fascinating state of Being, which human language completely fails to portray. Embodied human life, magnified a hundredfold in awareness, in intellectual acumen, and in the intensity of higher emotions would still fall short of the exaltation and exhiliration experienced in the beatific state.

This ravishment of the soul is mentioned by St. Macarius of Egypt in one of his Homilies: "And it comes to pass that, having been without leisure all the day, in this one hour he gives himself to prayer, and his inner man is rapt, in prayer, in the immeasurable depth of the other world, in such sweetness that his mind is far away, being soft and carried thither, so that at that time oblivion comes into his mind because it has been filled up and taken captive by divine and heavenly things, carried to the infinite and incomprehensible, to things so wonderful that they may not be expressed by human speech; thus, in that hour he prays and says: 'Would that my soul had gone forth together with the prayer.' When once through prayer or meditation or by merely evoking the image of Divinity the soul enters into communion with the Ineffable, it is drawn deeper and deeper with irresistible power until, in the highest stage, one can say with

Shams-i-Tabriz that being now devoid of all distinctions and free of the chains that bind it to the earth, it becomes so completely identified with the Over-Self that no distinction becomes possible. The individual then, torn from the anchor of corporeal selfhood, oblivious of the world and its problems, plunges into the Infinite, like a raindrop falling into the sea."

Mystical experience should not be viewed in isolation for any group of people, nor from the point of view of any particular faith, but rather, as a phenomenon of a universal character about the nature of which we are still in the dark. There is no fundamental difference between the pattern of the genuine mystical state experienced three thousand years ago, during the Vedic period, and that of today. It sounds paradoxical but it is true that, instead of an advancement in keeping with the improvement in the general intellectual level of mankind there has been regression in this direction, and in spite of the fact that the thirst for it continues unabated, the number of those who in recent times secured the supreme blessing of a mystical contact with the Divine has dwindled from that which prevailed during ancient or even medieval times. If the mystical experience betokens in reality a face-to-face encounter with Divinity or direct contact with universal consciousness, can there be anything more interesting and more important from the point of view of human aspirations than this for the attention and study of the human mind? That the quest has not been taken up in a serious way is a clear indication of the fact that either the phenomenon is not considered genuine by those competent to judge or for certain reasons no importance is attached to it.

Whatever the reason, viewed in the light of the facts mentioned in this volume, mystical experience of the right kind presents a problem which far exceeds in importance most other problems that engage the attention and consume the labor of countless painstaking investigators today. Because of its association with religion and the fact that the majority of those who earnestly strove for it in the past did so under the belief that the disciplines

undertaken or the austerities undergone provided the only way
to reach God, or to gain release from the cycle of births and
deaths in a tormenting world, mysticism, regarded as the crowning achievement of faith, became inextricably mingled with the
myths and superstitions of the various creeds, from which position
it has not been extricated so far. Even where a mystic, or a group
of mystics, raised a cry of revolt against the tenets or dogmas of
a particular religion or creed, there came into existence a new
faith with its own set of rituals and dogmas, which in the course
of time became as rigid and as unprogressive as the ones they had
replaced. Some of them, carried away by the stupendous nature
of their visions, identified themselves completely with what they
thought was God or the Absolute, relegating the world and every
human problem to a position of utter insignificance, unworthy
of attention from one blessed with the supreme happiness of
union with the Divine. This attitude of mind in the case of the
overzealous and the ignorant could not but lead to extremes: to
the negation of the world and its problems; to the neglect of the
body and the needs of the flesh; to excessive self-denial, self-
torture, and self-mortification; to distaste for life; to perversion
and distortion of the intellect; and last, but not the least, to an
obsessive preoccupation with the other world characterized by
fantasy and delusive states of the mind.

It is a fact of history that during the millenniums, beginning
about two thousand years before the birth of Christ, there appeared from time to time, in different parts of the world, specially gifted individuals who boldly proclaimed their connection
with a superearthly Fount of Intelligence and, by their extraordinary utterances and writings, their high ethical standards and
their intellectual attributes, proved their assertions to the satisfaction of the multitudes who followed them, leaving a mark on
history which is as fresh today as it was in their own time. They
present an enigma which even in this age of high intellectual
and scientific achievement still stands unsolved. They are the
founders of Yoga and every spiritual discipline, common or

esoteric, known to man. Almost all these illustrious personages had certain common characteristics that will be discussed later in this volume, and almost all of them had visionary experiences which guided them in creating unprecedented waves of enthusiasm among the people of their country and time for the attainment of spiritual ideals which were explained to them. As will be clarified later, the only rational explanation to account for this thus far inexplicable phenomenon lies in the admission that the human body has a still untapped reservoir of psychic energy and the human brain a hidden potentiality which, though dormant in the bulk of the race, somehow became active in these extraordinary men.

Once this is conceded, a ray of light begins to appear in the hitherto impenetrable darkness that surrounds mystical phenomena. The varied nature of the visionary experience, the variation in the degree of responsiveness in differently constituted individuals, the existence of the faculty in some from birth, and the need for employment of diverse methods, according to the psychophysiological condition of each individual, now stand partially explained. It becomes apparent that in dealing with the so-called supernatural phenomena and religious genius which have been an incomprehensible feature of civilization, almost from its very birth, we are not stepping out into a weird, uncanny world where the solid earth is left completely behind, nor are we entering into the domain of a capricious God or any other spiritual entity who bestows enlightenment on only those selected few, who sing His praises while mortifying themselves, and who keeps the rest in utter darkness of the spirit, but that here, as elsewhere in the sphere of biology, we are confronted by a yet incomprehensible law of nature and a still undiscovered vital mechanism in the human body which are at the root of this great mystery. This law and this power mechanism must have, like other aspects of nature, some definite aim in view. Considering the fact that all those extraordinary spiritual men and women who had this power center active from birth or who succeeded in stirring it to activity, possessed almost invariably exceptional powers of mind and spirit, it becomes clear without a shadow of doubt that the aim of this mysterious mechanism is the upgrading of human consciousness toward a summit about which we can only guess at present.

Viewed in the right perspective the mystic bears a message of tremendous import for all mankind. He is not the passive introvert or inert visionary sunk in his own delusions and lost to the world, as some people take him to be, nor is he doomed to be a recluse, abstaining from all the pleasures of life, as the religious-minded usually picture him or wish him to be. But he is the still imperfect forerunnner of the man to come, the ancestor of the future progeny, naturally endowed with a consciousness of the transcendent type, which the mystic experiences only rarely for brief durations with unutterable rapture, and finds it impossible to portray. He is the sef-controlled seer, idealized in the Upanishads and the Gita, rapt in the contemplation of the inner universe of Being, calm and serene, who has overcome passion and lust, and who performs all his duties in a spirit of dedication, not only for his own welfare but also for that of the world. He is the industrious, self-sacrificing savant, urgently needed in our day, calm and contented, who probes into the mysteries of nature to find something of advantage for the well-being of the race, who has solved the problem of his own being and gained access to the higher strata of life. He represents, in short, the cream of mankind in the near future, the leader of thought and the ruler of nations, who experiences the Transcendent, and, fortified with supernal wisdom, thus acquired, with coordinated effort brings peace and order in the present ill-managed, lust-ridden, passion-ruled world.

This vision of mystics of the future, resulting in a spiritually dominated, intellectual age, may appear unreal, exaggerated, or even fantastic to the rationalists, who see no possibility of such a drastic change in the nature of man, always under the subjugation of his instincts. For even those who believe in spiritual unfoldment and the existence of divine potentialities in man, the advent of a really great mystic is a rare occurrence, and the idea that a mystic hierarchy would ever come into being or, even if it did, would devote itself to the affairs of the world in the same manner as normal individuals do, may seem too utopian to be true. But seen dispassionately in the context of history, and in isolation from the agnostic trends of the day, a contrary view would be even more unrealistic and more at variance with the actual lessons of the past. Can there be any denial of the inviolable position that, all through the past, the greatest revolutions in human thought and human social orders were effected neither by men in power nor by those in possession of high intellectual endowments, divorced from the spiritual, but by those who had a powerful mystical streak in their composition? Do not the ideas of Yajnavalkya, Moses, Buddha, the other seers of the Upanishads, the prophets of the Old Testament, Socrates, Plato, Christ, Muhammad, Shankara, and others, all of them mystics of the highest order, still dominate the world? The upheavals caused by Darwin, Marx, Freud, and others in this age were not greater. The materialistic and mechanical view of life and mind which their ideas profess, lacks proof and has still to pass the acid test of time.

The issue has been touched in passing to bring into relief the decisive role played by mystics in molding the race and in shaping the course of history. It will be discussed in detail elsewhere to show that no great gulf intervenes between a top-rank intellectual and a visionary, and that the irreverent attitude of many present-day intellectuals toward religion, and the idea of hidden spiritual potentialities in men, originates from a skeptical materialistic tendency of our time. The main factors that have contributed to the creation of an atmosphere of doubt, even mistrust, toward religion and the Beyond are, first, that religion because of the generally dogmatic attitude of its exponents has not been able to keep pace with the advance in material science, and, second, because the leaders of spiritual thought fail to demonstrate the validity of their ideas and beliefs to the satisfaction of an unconvinced mind. If five hundred years before the birth of Christ, Gautama, the Buddha, had the intellectual acumen to find fault with the Vedas and to reject the metaphysical speculations of the Upanishads, which have an appeal for the erudite even today, how much more powerful must be the tendency in the modern intellectual, well aware of the recent revolutionary discoveries of science, and, at the same time, knowing the inanities, incredible beliefs, and irrational dogmas contained sometimes in the Scriptures of all religions and other books of faith, to harbor doubts and misgivings in regard to the religious doctrines and practices to which he is asked to conform implicitly, without criticism or questioning.

Modern man, layman or specialist, is hardly prepared to accept that, at present, the dubiously regarded mystical state is the most exalted and most productive condition of the human mind. He still has to understand that the veneration commanded by men belonging to this category is not an accident or a creation of the visionaries themselves in order to gain a position of eminence, but the outcome of a deeply rooted urge in human beings to show respect to one naturally endowed with a lofty attribute of the human mind necessary for the evolution of the race. Nor has he any inkling of the fact that this singular state of heightened perception can confer on those who attain to it such extraordinary powers of the spirit and mind as can prove of inestimable value in guiding mankind through the dangers of an uncontrolled technology and the hazards of a nuclear armament race. The ecstatic is the man par excellence, fashioned by nature to serve as a model for the multitudes, striving for happiness in a world still shrouded in darkness concerning the ultimate aim of human existence. If it is accepted that the transcendent consciousness, exhibited by many a prophet and seer of the past, is but a token of the lofty mental and spiritual outfit that will be the common heritage of the future man, the towering heights to which the outstanding personalities of the future will attain cannot even be imagined at present.

To avoid any ambiguity about the position presented in this volume, it is necessary to explain that the term *mystic,* as used here, includes every category of those men who, in one way or another, gain access to a transhuman state of consciousness and, by their own example and precept, furnish irrefutable evidence of extraordinary spiritual powers and intellectual gifts. The importance of this class of men, which includes all the well-known prophets, sages, and seers of the past, because of their exceptional talents, was thoroughly recognized in ancient times. The tragedy is that, on account of a grave misconception, widely prevalent in our time, namely, that man can know all that is worth knowing only by his intellect, people at large are under the impression that in temporal affairs a visionary is often out of place. The consequences of this misconception are obvious. Modern man still fails to make use of the spiritual potential present in him and depends too much on his intellect even in matters that are beyond its ken. The result is that, with all the amenities and luxuries provided by science, he lacks the possession of that peace and repose which are necessary for a fully satisfying and happy life. The lack of spiritual fulfillment in turn drives him to the use of undesirable surrogates, to alcohol, to drugs, to insatiable thirst for wealth and power, to sexual hyperaesthesia, and to other unsavory practices and occupations in order to appease the unassauged natural hunger in his mind.

With the recognition of the important role performed by the prophet and the seer in ancient times, numerous methods were devised by different people to attain the exceptional states of mind peculiar to them. The thirst for the fulfillment of spiritual ambitions or the desire for magical powers or psychic gifts provided the incentives for such arduous undertakings. The most elaborate system of tried practices and disciplines employed for this purpose in any country is provided by Yoga. Keeping in view the surpassing nature of the metamorphosis that has to be effected, and the extraordinary results that flow out of it in the case of successful initiates, it is no wonder that Yoga was always surrounded by a halo that has persisted to this day. Only the

general ignorance about the extraordinary nature of the alteration in the personality of the seeker keeps the modern intellectual
from becoming an ardent admirer of the system. At the present
moment the usual run of people who take to Yoga, apart from
the wholly devoted ascetic class, are those who, in addition to
their normal avocations, practice it as a subsidiary effort either
to gain psychic powers or success in their worldly ambitions or
to acquire peace of mind amid the distracting conflicts of a competitive life. In some cases the aim is transcendence, or rapport
with Divinity. A vast majority of the seekers of all these categories,
it can be readily observed, are of average and sometimes even
below average mental capacity. Many of them lack those attributes of character and that tenacity of purpose which are essential
for success in this extraordinary enterprise.

The doctrine of *kundalini,* the principal lever used in every
form of Yoga, holds hidden beneath a large mass of mysterious
formulas, strange practices, and rigid disciplines, inextricably involved in mythical verbiage, one of the greatest secrets of nature
known to man. As already mentioned the term *Yoga,* employed
in this volume, refers to all the methods that are known or that
will be known in any part of the world, which are effective in
leading people to supersensory states of consciousness and not
merely to conventional systems of Yoga. In this broad sense Yoga
is pregnant with a promise and a hope that far exceeds the highest expectations which its most enthusiastic adherents hold at
present. Yoga provides the only possible bridge between the
visible world and the unseen, the only ladder to reach the glorious heights of self-knowledge, the only method to remedy the
congenital defects of the brain or hereditary organic flaws of the
body, and the only way to determine the direction of human
evolution and the course of conduct men must follow to conform
to it. The usual benefits associated with Yoga—peace of mind,
transcendence, psychic gifts, and physical health—comprise but
a fraction of the immense possibilities that it holds. The reason
is simple. In his present way of life, man utilizes only a small

part of the psychic force residing in his body. The whole gamut of human progress achieved to this day, culminating in the visit to the moon, has been accomplished with the expenditure of this small amount of naturally available psychic energy, augmented from time to time in a few individuals by a trickle from the unused, hidden reservoir. Known spiritual prodigies and outstanding men of genius who, were they fashioned in a different way, could have utilized more of this psychic energy. They constitute the wellsprings from which the first tiny rivulets of original thought, both material and spiritual, flowed forth to mingle together and become a gradually widening and swiftly flowing stream with the subsequent small additions made by diligent men from the grateful multitudes.

Our aim in extending the sphere of Yoga to include every healthy and systematic aspect of religious endeavor is to focus attention on this issue of paramount importance, from both the physical and the spiritual points of view, that all the phenomena associated with religion, Yoga and the occult, of every shade and shape, spring from the possibility existing in the human organism, to alter the output of psychic energy under certain conditions, leading to a phenomenal transformation of the inner man. In its more pronounced forms the transformation may lead to a state of unimaginable glory, to the ascent of consciousness from the narrow periphery of a gloomy basement to the breathtaking pinnacle of universal Consciousness, for the first time made cognizant of its own unbounded proportions and immortal nature. The first impact of this stupendous vision on the seers is formidable, and it is no wonder that, under the stress of the flood of emotion experienced at the breathtaking spectacle, some of them at once faint away. This glorious consummation of spiritual effort, though rare, has been achieved time after time by earnest seekers of all epochs and countries. The transformation can become a permanent possession of an individual, resulting in a life of such fulfillment, peace, and beatitude as one can only associate with the godlike denizens of a glorious paradise.

The tendency to divide mystical phenomena into several arbitrary compartments and to extol this compartment or that, according to one's choice or inclination, springs from the fact that a high degree of ignorance still prevails about the basic factor responsible for them. Although, from the human point of view, there is no fundamental difference between Western mysticism, Sufism, Taoism, or Yoga, there is a general tendency, sometimes even among the intellectuals, to treat them as separate and distinct from each other. The main reason responsible for this uncalled-for discrimination probably lies in the fact that as, in the main, mystical experience is associated with the various religions and cults, the common strongly marked tendency that has persisted unaltered from very ancient times to differentiate among creeds has naturally been extended to the sphere of mystical phenomena also. The wonder is that although no distinction is made in the phenomenon of genius, and all talented men who had this heaven-bestowed spark in them, belonging to any country and epoch, are grouped under one category, irrespective of their faith or of the fact that they were born in the East or the West, the gifted mystics, who were equally the recipients of a heaven-granted extraordinary faculty, and, in the same way, are the common asset of all mankind, are nevertheless divided into groups and categories or differentiated according to the faith which they profess.

The subject is too vast to be dealt with here and will be discussed in detail elsewhere. It is enough to mention that all human beings, belonging to any racial group or to any part of the earth, have similar psychic and physiological reactions, the same emotions and passions, identical symptoms in bodily disease and mental disorder and, above all, the same construction of the various organs, the nervous system, and the brain. Yet some of the prevalent ideas, especially among the religious-minded and the credulous in respect to their approach to the Divine and the Transcendent, men, belonging to different faiths and different schools of spiritual discipline, are differentiated and regarded in dissimilar ways, and are, to say the least, infantile. They would have long since been labeled as blatantly ridiculous, but for the fact that they hold a large section of the believers still in their grip. If mystical experience is rooted in reality and is not merely a dream-like condition of the mind, it must have a common basis, run a uniform course and have a uniform symptomatology and climax for all men, perhaps with slight modifications due to temperamental and constitutional differences, as every other psychic manifestation in human beings. It must be subservient to a law or several laws, and must constitute an activity for which provision already exists in the human organism. It can in no case be an arbitrary excursion of the human mind into unknown regions of consciousness, engineered by man himself, without any legal sanction from Nature or from God.

The beatific vision cannot be a vision of God or union with Brahman, the Absolute, for the simple reason that the mental equipment of man and the consciousness that filters through it are too fragile and too dim, not even comparable to the faint glimmer of a tiny glowworm in an ocean of darkness, to have the capacity to apprehend, or to commune with, the Almighty Creator of this staggering universe. Considering the fact that consciousness exhibits itself on earth in an innumerable variety of forms, from the infinitesimal sentience of a cell to the flood of awareness in man, are we certain that no higher state of consciousness is possible on our globe and does not exist in any other part of the universe? If we are not sure of it, how can we then presume that man has attained the highest summit of knowledge and touched the border from where the exclusive conscious domain of God begins? It might be that what mystical experience represents, and what Yoga signifies, is the acquisition of or contact with a higher plane of consciousness, toward which mankind is slowly but inexorably evolving in a manner unknown to the scholars of this age. The transition from this state to the higher plane of consciousness might signify an ascent no less striking and no less wonderful than was the ascent from the anthropoid ape to man. All prophets, mystics, and seers as also those individuals (for instance Wordsworth) who had such experience without any specific religious discipline, might have had brief, long, or even permanent contacts with this higher plane of Being, which would seem as wonderful and as breathtaking as a sudden ascent to the level of human consciousness, with all its universe of thought and imagination, might have had for an ape.

This might be the explanation for all the supernatural and mystical phenomena exhibited, whether as an inborn gift or acquired with some kind of discipline, from the dawn of reason to the present day. The explanation is not offered in a spirit of arrogance, nor as an infallible conclusion communicated by a supernatural source, but in all humility as a humble contribution to knowledge from one who has undergone the experiences, from the simple to those of a high order, witnessing many of the phases and objectively studying his own mental conditions and reactions for decades before deciding to place the results of his observation before the world—not for instant acceptance or outright rejection but for study and investigation. Many difficulties will crop up in the unqualified acceptance of this view from both religion and science. The present work does not provide the scope for a discussion of the many implications of this view nor of objections likely to be raised.

The idea that in the ecstatic state of *samadhi,* the mystic or yogi does not behold the Creator or the Absolute need not cause a shock to the religious-minded. In fact, a contrary view would be even more sacrilegious for the reason that it is nothing short of presumption on the part of man, with all his frailities and limited mental equipment, to suppose that he has reached the summit of evolution and there are now no intermediary stages of perfection and intelligence between him and the Almighty Author of the universe. The mystics and Yoga saints themselves are divided over this important issue. From our present-day knowledge of the extent of the universe and the insignificant position occupied by earth, it is more difficult to maintain that in the unitive state the contemplative apprehends, beholds, or becomes identified with the unimaginably powerful Lord of this creation, the sole Support of countless suns and planets and the Refuge of countless forms of life throughout the universe, than to aver that the mystic state, or *turiya,* represents but another step on the ladder of evolution, raising man to a higher stratum of consciousness, with a tremendous enhancement in his powers of observation and with new channels of perception not exhibited by normal consciousness. The first transformation effected on his entry to this stratum is that he may become acutely aware of an all-knowing and all-pervasive state of Being, which may project itself on his perceptive faculty with or without a bodily form, entirely unlike anything known on earth. Whatever the nature of the vision or of the transformation witnessed in oneself, the unique, supernormal nature of the experience is unmistakable. The visionary now in touch with the stupendous, indescribable world of consciousness, interprets it as a contact with an almighty, omniscient Divine Being and may have the realization that the Being has entered into him or that he is one with It.

In actual fact what he perceives is himself with a highly enhanced supersensory form of awareness, in contact now with the subtle universe of consciousness that was previously impervious to his inner vision. The ecstasies and entrancements, the confusions and contradictions, the varied sensations and surmises, the diverse nature of the visions and values and the divergent interpretations placed on the experience by the mystics themselves, that present a dilemma for scholars, could never be a characteristic of the unitive state were it, in the real sense, a union between the Almighty and man. Anomalies, conflicts, and variations occur because the brain has to adjust itself to the new development. As the power of adjustment varies with different people and the experience is affected by their constitution, temperament, thoughts and fancies, religious and social environments, individual idiosyncrasies and suggestions of preceptors, it is no wonder that the whole phenomenon, at the present stage of our knowledge of it, presents such a host of variations and incongruities that the bewildered intellect finds it difficult to assign its origin to the same cause. This does not mean that by this transformation man does not rise nearer to Divinity or that he does not develop divine attributes to attain this sublime state. He certainly rises higher in the scale of evolution, coming into possession of new talents and powers, with new channels of cognition and a new vision of the universe and his own life, and he surely needs an all-round ethical development as a precondition to the ascent. But he is still far, far from God or the Absolute and even the apex of his own evolution. In the most perfect cases he can become a superman, an arhat, a Buddha, a prophet, a savior, a *jivan-mukhta* (one liberated in life), an adept, or an illumined sage.

How does this incredible metamorphosis come about? What invisible psychic forces, activated by devotion, passionate longing, austerity, meditation, or other practices, are generated and come to the rescue of the soul to release it from its prison and raise it to a state of unparalleled glory and universal being? What carries it to the uttermost limits of knowledge and existence, so that nothing greater or more sublime can be known or experienced in human life? It cannot be, as is commonly supposed, an external agency, propitiated or invoked by these practices, which comes to the aid of the devotee to lift him up from darkness into light or from human to Cosmic Consciousness. What is more probable and more in accordance with the methods employed by nature, is that there must be something already provided in the soul-body combination we call man, still a source of wonder and mystery to the learned, which is capable of remolding the whole organism with the help of a still unidentified Source of Energy, hidden in the depths of the body, which is at the root of all the transcendent phenomena exhibited by men. This something must also be the hidden power behind Yoga, the vast reservoir of psychic energy, designed by nature for the evolution of man which, when channeled in the right direction, can work miracles with his body and the brain to infuse him with a new life and a new consciousness. There is irrefutable evidence to show that this power mechanism has been known and manipulated in different ways to gain magical powers or transcendent states of consciousness from very ancient times, but so far no attempt has been made to dissociate it from the miraculous and the supernatural and to bring it within the orbit of a demonstrable natural law governing the evolution of the human race.

3

Kundalini, Fact and Fiction

The general idea prevailing about *Kundalini,* in both the East and the West, is of a mysterious and fabulous power lying dormant in men, which, when roused to activity, can confer amazing psychic gifts and transhuman states of consciousness on the successful initiates. The belief is current in India and elsewhere that those, in whom the energy vivifies the seventh center in the brain, are transmogrified and attain unlimited dominance over the forces of nature. This belief is fostered by the high claims made in the ancient literature on Kundalini-Yoga about the infinite possibilities for the elevation and deification of those who propitiate this divine power. The ascent of *Kundalini* from *Cakra** to *Cakra** is attended, it is said, with progressively increasing psychic powers until in the seventh center the mortal becomes one with the supreme Reality, or Lord Shiva, the Creator, Preserver, and Destroyer of the three worlds. The Yogi, it is averred, gains unlimited powers of domination over men, fascination for women, and sovereignty over the forces of nature. Thus in Mahanirvana

---

* Cakra: In Yogic parlance Cakra signifies a center of psychic force, said to be existing on the cerebro-spinal axis, beginning from Muladhara, or root-support center, at the base of the spine. The number of Cakras, as now generally held, is six through which Kundalini rises on its ascent to Sahasrara in the crown of the head. In the ancient texts these centers are depicted as being circular in formation.

Tantra (vii. 39,40,41,50) it is said that he who worships the Adya-Kali (*kundalini*) Mistress of the three worlds "Becomes in learning like Brhaspati (the Guru of the Celestials), in wealth like Kubera (the god of riches). . . . Men bow with respect at the mere mention of his name. The eight *siddhis* (i.e., the power to become exceedingly large or extremely small or light as a feather, to float in space, or to become invisible to sight, or to enter the bodies of others, to be clairvoyant, clairaudient, or to have domination over all the forces, etc.), he looks upon as mere bits of grass."

There is no end to the *siddhis* (supernatural powers) promised in the ancient writings to those who succeed in awakening *kundalini*. Thus in Ṣat-Cakra-Nirupana (vs. 21) it is said: "By meditating on this Navel Lotus (*Nabhi-Padma*) the power to destroy and create (the world) is acquired. Vani, (the goddess of speech) with all the wealth of knowledge ever abides in the lotus of his face." Again in verse 31: "He who has attained complete knowledge of the Atman (Brahman) becomes, by constantly concentrating his mind (*citta*) on this Lotus, a great sage (*Kavi*), eloquent and wise, and enjoys uninterrupted peace of mind. He sees the three periods (past, present, and future), and becomes the benefactor of all, free from disease and sorrow, long-lived, and, like Hamsa, the destroyer of endless dangers."

The possibility offered by the Tantric Sadhana to gain longevity, health, and miraculous powers seems to have been exploited to the full by the ancient exponents of the system to attract the attention of the multitudes and to gain followers for the cult. The promise of these extraordinary achievements was not extended to men only but also to women. Thus it is stated in Hathayoga-Pradipika (iii.102): "The woman who (with the practice of Vajroli Mudra), applying suction with her (female genital organ) directs the reproductive secretion in the upper direction (i.e., draws it into the head), becomes a Yogini with the power to know the past, present, and future and to float in air." I have quoted these passages to show that what many modern seekers expect from Yoga, in the wildest flights of their fancy, is already offered in the old manuals and, according to some of them, can be had merely for the asking.

It is easy to see that the achievements are highly exaggerated, a common tendency among ancient authors, and that there is not only no end to the glowing promises held out but also undisguised contradictions in the statements. For while some emphasize lifelong effort and hard discipline to gain the favor of the goddess to achieve this or that *siddhi,* others consider mere proficiency in but one asana or in some single Pranayama or mere repetition (*japa*) of a *mantra* sufficient to gain the most rewarding supernatural gifts. The pity is that no attempt has been made to separate the chaff from the wheat, and in the current literature on the subject only the old rituals, down to the most obscene ones, the old practices, formulas, and promises are being interminably repeated without any effort at clarification to show what deserves credence and what should be rejected as mere superstition or exaggeration, impossible of acceptance in this rational age. It can be confidently asserted that there is a solid core of truth in the assertions of the ancient authors which has been so exaggerated and embellished that a doubt is cast over the whole system. What is more important, from the present-day point of view, is that this solid core has the unique possibility of providing empirical evidence for its support to the satisfaction of even the most skeptical intellects. The aim of this work is to lay open this possibility by subjecting the ancient as well as the current ideas and theories about Kundalini-Yoga to a critical analysis in the light of modern knowledge about the human mind and body. The attitude adopted in India during the past several centuries, in respect to the ancient treatises on Yoga, has been and still is one of uncritical acquiscence under the impression that the authorities are too lofty and the subject too sacrosanct to be critically examined in this profane age. This supine attitude has done no good to anyone but, on the contrary, has resulted in pushing into oblivion one of the greatest discoveries ever made by man, for the simple reason that the discovery at present is represented in a manner which is repugnant to commonsense.

It is unfortunate that there is no book on Kundalini-Yoga, written by a modern intellectual, well acquainted with the present-day concepts of science, based on his own experience of the divine power. Most of the writers on the subject either merely copy the ancient books or try to interpret the writings in the light of their own spiritual and metaphysical ideas. The nature of the mysterious force has not been defined or elucidated in a rational way in any treatise ancient or modern. The general impression about the awakening among those interested in the subject is, therefore, of a sudden leap from the visible world of rigid cause and effect to a transmundane state of existence where everything becomes possible; a dangerous position in this age of reason, fostered by writers with a predilection for the supernatural and the uncanny for whom every word of the ancient manuals has the weight of a gospel. Except for the nature of nerve energy, which carries out the multifarious activities of the body in a most amazing manner and every moment flashes thousands of signals from the various organs and limbs to the brain and vice versa, modern physiology has drawn an almost complete picture of the human frame, its organs and their functions, and no obscure region or crevice has been omitted, save for some portions of the brain and the spinal cord, about which knowledge is still extremely meager. There is apparently no visible biological device in the body capable of generating a spiritual energy of the fabulous kind, as is mentioned in the literature on the subject. The organs at the base of the spine are the rectum and the sexual parts and their functions are well known. How can this area, the skeptics may reasonably ask, be the seat of a magical force which can effect such a radical change in the human system as to make it capable of superhuman feats?

The ancient exponents of this Yoga meet this obvious objection by the argument that *kundalini*, in the wider sense of the term, is the Cosmic Life Energy or *Prana-Shakti*, the source of all the phenomena of life in the universe, and that in the microcosm, represented by man, She (*Shakti*), in a corresponding form, resides at the base of the spine in the form of a serpent, coiled three and a half times, closing with her mouth the lower entrance to the passage leading to the abode of Shiva or Brahman in the crown of the head. In average men and women She lies asleep, or in a static form, i.e., coiled, conditioning the human consciousness so that, forgetful of its own divine, immortal nature, it allows itself to be caught in the toils of the constantly changing, phenomenal world. When roused to activity with appropriate methods She, like a streak of lightning, darts through the *Suṣumna,* clearing the darkness that holds the embodied spirit bound to the earth. According to the concept of the ancient authorities, therefore, *kundalini* is divine in nature, the superintelligent creative aspect of Lord Shiva, the Creator, Sustainer and Destroyer of the world, one with Him in the unmanifested state; but while He even in the manifested state continues to bide without any change or modification, unaffected by the emergence and dissolution of the Cosmic hosts, She, as the Creatrix, manifests Herself both as the created objects and the energy that sustains them. "She is the Omnipotent Kala who is wonderfully skillful to create," says Sat-Cakra-Nirupana (vs. 12), "and is subtler than the subtlest. She is the receptacle of that continuous stream of ambrosia which flows from the Eternal Bliss. By Her radiance it is that the whole of this universe and this Cauldron is illumined."

In fact for Her devotees She has the same absolute position and the same unlimited powers as are associated with God, Isvara, Allah, or Jehovah by the religious-minded. With such a conception of the divine energy (*kundalini*) it is no wonder that the ancient authors have been most lavish in their praises and exhausted the power of their genius in investing her with all the attributes and all the powers—Omnipresence, Omnipotence, Omniscience—befitting the Creatrix and the absolute Ruler of the world. The reason for assigning an almost divine position to the Gurus who succeed in establishing rapport with Her and investing them with all the virtues and unrestricted supernatural powers, befitting those who have won the favor of the Almighty Controller of the universe, thus becomes apparent. It is the same old idea, expressed in a different way, that by propitiating the Almighty, Unseen Power behind the Cosmos through austerity, worship, and various other forms of spiritual discipline, one can attain the lofty position of a direct inner contact with Him, paving the way to superhuman attributes and supernatural powers, which is prevalent in almost all the existing great religions of mankind and which acted as a powerful guiding factor in primitive cults and religious practices as well. In the microcosmic form the all-powerful Creative Energy (*shakti*) is symbolized in the form of a coiled serpent, i.e., in a state of inaction, residing at the base of the spine in the human body. The aim of Kundalini-Yoga is to awaken the serpent and to force her, stage by stage, to ascend the spinal canal, known as *susumna,* until She reaches the seat of Shiva in the highest center in the brain. This ascent, it is stated, takes years to accomplish, though in exceptional cases only a short time, constantly attended by divine manifestations. At each of the five lower *cakras,* or lotuses, the ascending *shakti* dissolves one of the five primordial elements of which the visible cosmos is constituted (namely, earth, water, fire, air and ether) into the basic substance, which is consciousness, until after dissolving the mind and ego, which are also the forms of primeval *shakti,* the liberated spirit finds itself in ecstatic union with the Eternal Conscious Reality to which it owes its being.

Many modern writers on the subject have taken the same line and ascribe the phenomena associated with *kundalini* to the existence of a cosmic, astral, etheric, or psychic force without any biological connection with the human body, much in the same fashion as has been done in the ancient treatises. They override the physiological objections to the existence of lotuses on the spinal cord, or of any structure in the flesh resembling a coiled serpent at the base of the spine, or of the other objects mentioned in the ancient books by saying that all these formations on the spinal cord and the brain, to which the ancient Scriptures refer with confidence, have no tangible physical reality, but exist in the astral body or the subtle sheath of *prana,* surrounding the physical frame. In the same manner the term *nadis,* frequently used in the treatises on Hatha Yoga, is held to signify subtle channels of psychic energy or invisible *prana* that have no identity with the network of nerves, veins, and arteries distributed over the whole body. There can be no denial of the fact that the potent pranic current generated by the body, on the awakening of *kundalini,* is of such a marvelous nature, and acts with such unerring precision and superhuman intelligence, that it reaches the province of the Divine; yet for all practical purposes and in all its physical and physiological bearings the foundation of the power firmly rests on the biological structure of the human frame. From the purely scientific view, therefore, some of the basic assumptions of Kundalini-Yoga have no existence in reality according to the interpretation put on the word *nadis* and *lotuses* by some modern authors. In other works, however, *nadis* are translated as arteries.

The *cakras* to which repeated reference is made by both ancient and modern writers and which, in fact, by constant use have become so familiar that the very name *cakra* has assumed the significance of *kundalini,* are held by some authorities to represent nerve plexuses of the central or autonomous nervous system, and by others as subtle vortices of *prana* energy, located at different places in the brain and the spinal cord, having no corporeal lineaments visible to the eye. They can be observed, they say, only with internal vision acquired when Kundalini is awakened. These vortices are said to exist in the form of lotuses with a specific number of petals in each. The lotus in the lowest or *muladhara cakra* has four petals; the next above it, *svadisthana,* six; the *manipura,* or navel plexus, ten; the next above *anahata* or heart center, twelve; the *visuddha,* or throat plexus, sixteen; the *ajna cakra,* or the lotus between the eyebrows, two; and the last, the *sahasrara,* is said to be a lotus with a thousand petals situated in the cerebrum.

The total number of petals in the six lotuses from the *muladhara* to *ajna cakra* is fifty, which corresponds to the number of letters in the Sanskrit alphabet. In fact, each petal of every lotus has a letter on it, which, all combined, form the Sanskrit alphabet or Verna-mala. In addition to the letters each lotus has a presiding *shakti,* or goddess, with a specific shape and color. The Buddhist Tantrics recognize only four *cakras,* or lotuses, beginning at the umblical cord and ending in the Usnisa-Kamla (lotus) in the head, corresponding to *sahasrara.* The other two correspond to the *anahata* and *visuddha* in the cardiac and laryngeal regions. In some ancient statues of Buddha the opened Usnisa-Kamala is depicted by a slight protuberance on the top of the head. The general impression prevailing at present that there are seven Cakras on the cerebro-spinal axis is of comparatively recent origin. In the early Upanishads only one, two, or three centers are mentioned, while in some texts dealing with *kundalini* ten, eleven, and even more *cakras* are described. The Brhadarnyka-Upanishad (2. 1. 19 and 4.2.3) mentions only the heart-center as the seat of origin of the *nadis* that carry *prana* energy to every part of the body. In his exposition of the Yoga Sutras of Patanjali, Vacaspati Misra (i. 36) makes mention of the lotus of the Heart and Susumna; and Patanjali himself (iii. 29) refers to *nabhi-cakra* as a center for concentration. The other *cakras* mentioned in Tantric texts are Yonisthana, Lalana, Manas, and Soma Cakras. According to Shiva-Samhita (ii. 28) besides the six Cakras there are five other centers with many names. In a comparatively recent Sanskrit work, Advaita Martanda, no less than twenty *cakras* are enumerated. Meditation on any one of the six Cakras, it is said, can lead to the arousal of *Kundalini.* Different psychic powers are associated with each *cakra.* The lotuses, the letters on their petals, the Bija Mantras, the presiding *Shaktis* with their appearance and accoutrements are clearly mentioned in the ancient texts, and vividly depicted on the illustrations drawn in ancient times. They present an intriguing and fascinating study that has largely contributed to arousing the curiosity of seekers about this form of Yoga from very ancient times to the present day.

The question that now arises is how far these descriptions of

Cakras, their lotuses, and other accessories correspond to reality and have a substratum of truth in them. To a scientific mind, acquainted with the anatomy of the human body, the diagrams and the descriptions would at first sight strike one as the products of a brain which, to say the least, has lost touch with actuality and lives in a fantastic realm of dreams. It would dismiss the whole subject as entirely unscientific and irrational, the fanciful creation of deluded anchorites or of unscrupulous charlatans to deceive the credulous. In fact, even in India, the Tantric rites and practices have been and are severely criticized by the followers of Vedic systems of ritual and worship. In view of this, it is not difficult to imagine how impossible it is for a modern informed mind to reconcile the descriptions of the ancient masters, relating to the *cakras* and the lotuses, with the characteristics of the cerebro-spinal system contained in modern texts on physiology. It is not, therefore, to be wondered that the Yoga, dealt with in the Tantras labors under a cloud, and that modern writings on the subject by adhering to ancient terminology and descriptions, instead of attempting to present this venerable system within the framework of modern knowledge, tend to render it more unintelligible and obscure.

In order to establish the existence of the power reservoir of *kundalini* on a scientific basis, acceptable to a strictly rational mind, it is absolutely necessary to explain the existing discrepancies in the accounts of different authors and to elucidate and reconcile the apparently fantastic and impossible assertions about the lotuses and the Cakras in order to clear the cobwebs that have grown around the subject in the course of the ages. The ancient, or the present, unrealistic mode of presentation of this Yoga might result in a progressively diminishing audience for some time to come, and help the writers to maintain the illusion among a sector of the credulous and uncritical seekers for the supernatural. But it can neither do any real service to this ancient system of religious discipline nor help to uncover the momentous discovery of the highest importance that lies concealed under the cloak of weird formulations, fantastic creations and mythical beings. Considering the general ignorance concerning the basic facts of physiology prevailing during the past, and the superstitious awe with which the inexplicable phenomena relating to the mind and body were regarded, even by the intelligent and the learned in ancient times, it is not surprising that the ancient masters created a whole host of divinities and strange formations in the body to account for the bewildering effects caused by *kundalini*. But now a rational explanation is unavoidable.

Before taking up the issue of lotuses, described in lavish detail, let us confine ourselves to the discussion of the presiding *shaktis* that pervade the *cakras* and are meticulously portrayed in the ancient texts. A mere glance at their names, *Dakini, Rakini, Kakini, Sakini, Lakini* and *Hakini,* is enough to convey to any discriminating intellect that the appellations are crudely fabricated and can only deceive the ignorant or the extremely credulous. No rational man can even for a moment accept the existence of supernatural beings with such a string of designations that cannot fail to strike even the least informed as being artificial and fictitious. Some modern writers have tried to interpret these *shaktis* in terms of particular nerves dominating the various plexuses. If this interpretation is accepted we will have to accept the same interpretation for the lotuses as well, and also for such other creations of the ancient masters as appear improbable and fantastic to the modern mind. The experts who witnessed the phenomenon in themselves, completely baffled by the strange effects and weird displays produced by the impact of the newly generated vital currents at the various nerve junctions on the spinal axis, could not but attribute the mysterious happenings to the agency of various supernatural entities whom they designated as *shaktis* in keeping with the conception that the human body and the whole Cosmos were the manifestation of an almighty divine Energy, *maha–shakti* or *parmeshvari*.

The association of the letters in the Sanskrit alphabet with the petals of the lotuses is another bald fact unacceptable to commonsense. If the lotuses exist, even on the psychic plane, it is incredible that heaven should have so arranged their petals as to correspond exactly to the number of letters used in the Sanskrit text. Whether they exist on the astral or the physical realm they could never be intended by nature to serve the purpose of one particular language to the exclusion of the others. There is no reason why the Chinese characters or Egyptian hieroglyphics or the cuneiform writing of the Sumerians or the script of the ancient inhabitants of the Indus Valley which are at least as old as Sanskrit, do not find any place on the lotuses, if they are really part and parcel of the human body, or even on the astral plane, an etheric or psychic counterpart of it, and not merely imaginary objects intended to convey some purpose about which we are in the dark at present.

The Bija-Mantras are no less inexplicable. The very nature of the sounds emitted by the *mantras, Ham, Vam, Yam, Lam, Tham,* etc., are a clear indication of the fact that they are fabricated and are as imaginary as the presiding *shaktis* and the letters of the alphabet. It is evident that when repeated interminably in a state of intense concentration, with diminished breathing and heart action, they can serve effectively, with their nasal intonation and monotonous sonority, to induce a state of quiescence preceding the state of trance. Monotonous sounds have been used from prehistoric times and are even now employed by hypnotists and teachers of the occult to induce somnambulistic conditions. In primitive societies, in all periods of history down to recent times, monotonous chanting and weird music have always been used to induce abnormal mental conditions and trancelike states in sensitive persons, susceptible to occult influences. The recitation of the Bijas or other Mantras, prescribed by the Guru, causes the same somnolent effect in the Sadhakas with a largely enhanced effect in combination with the other mental and physical exercises enjoined. It is easy to see that the Mantras of the class *Aim, Hrim, Krom, Srim Svaha,* or *Hrim, Srim, Krim, Parameshvari Svaha* (Mahanirvana Tantra vi. 72-74 and 82) or others used in Tantric Sadhna are definitely of the hypnotic type.

It is obvious that the lotuses, the presiding *Shaktis,* the letters of the alphabet, the Bija-Mantras and other objects, as well as the diagrammatic formations meticulously described in the ancient manuals and shown graphically in the illustrations, have no real existence and are the mental creations of the masters to provide a physical representation for their teaching as well as to invest it with a certain amount of mystery, solemnity, and awe —all of them necessary ingredients of every effective religious practice and discipline. It has to be remembered that the system of Kundalini-Yoga is of great antiquity, probably extending to an epoch antecedent even to the Indus Valley civilization. It is a well-known fact that up to comparatively recent times even physicians had fantastic notions about blood, phlegm, menses, and the like, as well as about the organs and their functions, and maladies were often attributed to the evil influence of spirits, demons, and other diabolic supernatural sources. The people often resorted to exorcism, spells, and charms or other magical cures for even the most dangerous and virulent diseases which modern rational methods of treatment are now slowly bringing under control. In such a milieu of ignorance and superstition, it is no wonder that fantastic stories were current about the phenomenon of *kundalini,* and that its exponents should themselves have weird notions about the mysterious power. They made use of Hermetic methods and cabalistic signs, and peopled the whole region, from the base of the spine to the crown of the head (in which the impact of the force is felt) with strange objects and supernatural entities to account for the unusual manifestations. What other reaction could be expected to a rare and mysterious biological phenomenon which, even in our age of progress, has not been identified as yet, and, when located, is very likely to prove a difficult problem for the most learned?

Modern authors have drawn from writings that are centuries old, dating back to times when the world was still shrouded in the gloom of ignorance and the people were much more in the grip of the uncanny and the supernatural. It is a testimony to the rarity of the phenomenon that, in recent times, no adept of this form of Yoga has appeared to recast the ancient treatises in order to bring them in line with the enormous advances made in psychology, physiology, and other branches of knowledge relevant to this subject. At the same time great credit is due to the ancient authors who, in spite of the handicaps under which they were laboring and the ignorance prevailing in their time, displayed a considerable knowledge of the nervous system, out of all proportion to the general level of the information available, acquired no doubt by observing internally the movements of the luminous currents released by an awakened *kundalini*.

For a manual suited to the level of knowledge of the present day it is necessary to clarify the position in respect to these imaginary descriptions of the ancient authors and to concentrate only on the scientific implications of the phenomenon. A modern aspirant, burdened with the conventional details, would not only find himself on the horns of a dilemma, unable to reconcile the fully substantiated and thoroughly investigated findings of anatomy with the strange objects and mysterious beings said to be residing at different places on the spinal cord, but also see his efforts to decipher these hieroglyphics turning into a will-o'-the-wisp chase which can lead him nowhere. For the ancient seekers, to whom the enterprise was the main object of life, a long course of instruction in the mysteries and intricacies of the esoteric system was necessary to keep them engaged, and to instill a sense of reverence for the teacher and the subject, making it necessary for the former to embellish it with mythical divinities and enigmatic figures in order to sustain the curiosity and interest of their disciples.

This brings us to the basic issue of the reality of the Cakras themselves. Divested of the imaginary embellishments, what remains are concentrations of nerves, having a circular formation. Here we tread on solid ground, verifiable in terms of our present knowledge of the human body. For at the places, where the Cakras are said to be located, there are thick clusters of intersecting nerves which become at once recognizable when the powerful stream of nerve energy, generated by *kundalini,* begins to circulate in the system. With a little more improvement in the delicate instruments that are now used to measure the electrical activity of the brain and the speed of nerve impulses, it might become possible at no distant date to detect variations in the quality and potency of nerve currents. When this comes to pass, the changes wrought in the nervous system by an active *kundalini* as well as the passage of the more potent current through the criss-crossing nerve junctions can be easily detected. Even at present more than sufficient evidence is furnished by the ancient writings, provided they are sanely interpreted, to show that, although the whole phenomenon is attributed to the activity of a superhuman power, the biological reactions that occur as a result of it are, to a large extent, understood and dealt with in proper ways in keeping with the level of knowledge of the times.

Some of the present-day exponents, unable to reconcile the lotuses and their accessories with the findings of modern physiology and caught in the labyrinth of ancient writings, interpret the term *nadis* as subtle channels of *prana,* different from nerves. They adopt a stand which is contradicted by the fundamental teaching of the Tantras themselves. All the disciplines of Kundalini-Yoga are directed towards Bhutta Shuddhi, i.e., for the purification of the five gross elements in the body. This purification can only be effected through the instrumentality of the bodily organs controlled by the nervous system and the brain. In fact, the whole armory of Hatha-Yoga practices—Posture, *Shatkarma,* Concentration, or *Pranayama*—is aimed to secure control or to improve the functions of the various organs with the ultimate object of gaining power over the vital processes of the body in order to force the arousal of the serpent power. When awakened, the live, pranic force, coursing through the nerves, effects the purification of the body and the transformation of the brain to make supersensory experience possible. When we readily acknowledge what is a matter of daily observation, that the spirit animating us, in spite of its divine nature, can act only on and by the body through the brain, the nervous system and the intricate complex of the biological organism, how can we then assume that any other divine agency can act on the same body directly, effectuating radical changes and transformations, without the agency of the brain, the nervous system or other vital organs? If *nadis* are merely incorporeal channels of *prana,* through what channel then do the changes and the manifestations in the body occur? In the light of these facts it is not only against the spirit of the ancient writings, but also against the dictates of common-sense and the highly scientific nature of this venerable system to invoke superphysical and unverifiable agencies to account for a phenomenon that can be explained in strictly rational terms.

In his exposition of the Yoga-Sutras of Patanjali (iii. 32) Vacas-pati-Mishra says that "the words (in the head) imply the tube (*nadi*), called *susumna,* and that Patanjali means *samyama* on that." The words 'in the head' clearly indicate a location for the tube *susumna,* which establishes its corporeal nature. This is confirmed in Katha-Upanishad (11.3.16) in these words: "The nerves of the heart are a hundred and one in number. Of them the one (*susumna*) passes through the head. Going up through that nerve one achieves immortality. The others that have different directions become the cause of death." Further confirmation comes from Brhadaranyaka-Upanishad (iv. 2.3): "And this human form that is in the left eye is his wife, Viraj (matter). This space that is within the heart is their place of union. The mass of blood which is in the heart is their food. What looks like a net within the heart is their covering. The nerve that rises upward from the heart is their passage for moving; it is like a hair split into a thousand parts. (Numerous) nerves (*nadis*) of this body called Hita, are rooted in the heart. It is through these that the essence of food passes when it moves. Hence the subtle body has finer food than the gross body." It is the nerves that extract the finer essence from the body which circulates as psychic and nerve energy in the system.

This biological essence or individual *prana* is the connecting link between the corporeal body and the incorporeal Cosmic Life-energy. Again the same Upanishad states (iv. 3. 20): "In a man are these nerves (*nadis*) called Hita, which are as fine as a hair split into a thousand parts, and full of white, blue, brown, green and red (serums). . . ." There can be no doubt that the reference is to the bodily nerves. It is no exaggeration to say that some of the nerve fibrils are as fine as the thousandth part of a hair. The colors are supposed to be due to the mixture of wind, bile, and phlegm in varying proportions, according to the prevalent notions of the time. Pancastavi (vs. 2) likens *kundalini* to the fine filament of the maidenhair fern, a very apt illustration for the slender nerve-fibers covering the human body. This view is again unequivocally confirmed by Hatha-Yoga-Pradipika (ii. 4) in these words "So long as *nadis* remain clotted with impurity the movement of *prana* does not occur through the middle passage (*susumna*) and so long as *prana* does not flow through *susumna* how can success attend the undertaking? In order to become affected by impurity the *nadis* must have a corporeal nature. *Pranayama* and other practices of Hatha-Yoga aim to remove this impurity.

Shiva-Samhita (2. 29,30,31,32) gives a graphic description of the anatomical arrangement of the nerves (*nadis*) which can leave no one in doubt about their physical character. In order to arrive at a correct evaluation of the accounts of the ancient authors it must be borne in mind that the descriptions cannot be as detailed and accurate as are contained in a modern manual of physiology for the reason that the structure of the body was an unfathomable mystery in their time, and though the pulse-beat was well known, the riddle of the flow of blood was still unsolved. Considered in the light of these facts this description of the nervous system is singularly informative. It says: "Other *nadis* (besides *susumna*) rising from muladhara spread to the tongue, penis, eyes, big toes, ears, abdomen, armpits, thumbs, and lower limbs, and terminate there. From these *nadis* by the process of ramification and branching there arise 350,000 *nadis* existing at their respective places.

All these vital nadis are efficient in carrying *prana* (from one part to the other) and by division and multiplication are spread all over the body." The view expressed by Arthur Avalon and others that *nadis* are subtle channels of pranic or vital energy is not thus borne out by the statements contained in the ancient treatises. Once it is admitted that the term *nadis* used by ancient writers refers to nerves present in our flesh and blood, there should come a change in the concept of Kundalini-Yoga, and the doctrine, coming down from the unverifiable planes of incorporeality, should touch the solid surface of earth as a verifiable biological phenomenon. All this possesses profound significance which will be explained elsewhere in this volume. Had the system of *kundalini* been elaborated by any other people independently, it is possible that they might have associated their own script with it in some way though not precisely in the same manner, as has been done in India. In order to clarify this rather cryptic statement it is enough to mention here that as Revelation and Genius proceed from an awakened *kundalini,* and language is the main channel for the expression of both, the association of the Sanskrit alphabet or, for that matter, of any other alphabet, with the other symbolic representations of the mysterious Force is, therefore, a perfectly natural process. Since this relationship, though well known to the ancient masters, has not been explicitly brought out in any ancient treatise, not one of the modern expositors of this Yoga, in spite of deep study and research, has been able to understand or explain its significance, which is of a paramount nature. The tendency to cover the science of life with a mantle of superstitious ritual, mythical personages, mysterious happenings and miraculous powers, representing an earlier stage in the development of the human mind, seriously retards instead of advancing, in this age of widespread knowledge and progress, the cause of this most important doctrine which rationally approached and critically examined can prove to be a veritable mine of surprises and new discoveries for both the seekers after God and the votaries of science.

It is a matter of common observation that we live in two worlds, one physical and the other spiritual. The visible universe and our bodies are made of this physical stuff, but our thoughts and consciousness are formed to be of an intangible substance about which, even in this era of phenomenal progress in knowledge, we as yet know next to nothing. This subtle world of thoughts, fancies and dreams is as basic a fact of our experience as the physical universe, and is decidedly nearer and more intimate to us than the latter. But it is so inextricably linked up with every cell and fiber of our flesh that it appears to be an inseparable product of our physical body. It is true that if consciousness and thought are self-existing substances, and not merely the products of cellular activity, they should have an independent existence as well as spheres of activity of their own, but viewed from our experience this holds true only in the abstract. For we never perceive consciousness or thought operative without the vehicle of flesh. It is precisely here that *kundalini* plays a decisive role. As if alive to human aspirations at a certain stage of intellectual development, far-sighted nature has planted a divine mechanism in the human body, which by effecting an alteration in the vital energy, or *prana,* feeding the brain, can bring the amazing universe of consciousness within the range of awareness of an awakened man.

The whole science of *kundalini* is based on the manipulation of *prana-vayu,* the nerve junctions (*cakras*), and the brain. *Vayu* in Sanskrit means *air* and the word is used with *prana* to denote its subtle nature. *Prana* and *vayu* are, sometimes, interchangeably used by the ancient authors to designate nerve energy or vital breath. Although *prana* is a self-existent substance, deathless and all-pervading, yet its manifestation in the bodies of terrestrial creatures is rigidly regulated by biological laws. In fact, the whole animal kingdom is the product of the activity of *prana* and the atoms of matter both combined. *Prana* is not something radically different from matter, but both are derivatives from the same basic substance, *para-shakti* or Primordial Energy. At the present

stage of our knowledge nothing would be more ridiculous than
to suppose that this combination of *prana* and matter which has
resulted in such marvelous organizations of living creatures, can
be so flimsy and unstable as to yield readily to the human will.
The impression prevailing in the minds of some people that a
few minutes' exercise of concentration can work miracles in
changing one's existing level of consciousness with the arrest of
prana and thought is, therefore, as correct as it would be to suppose that repeated light hammer-blows dealt to a metal can lead
to the release of atomic energy. An overhauling of the entire
human body is necessary to effect a radical transformation in its
consciousness from the normal to the supersensory level. This is
the reason why real success in Yoga is so very rare. The actual
position is that a large proportion of even those who take to the
study and practice of Yoga are, not infrequently, themselves
ignorant of the Herculean nature of the enterprise that confronts
them, and the marvelous transformation of consciousness that
can occur by this means.

The ancient writers have made no secret of this formidable
task, impossible of achievement through human efforts alone.
Only because nature has provided a contrivance in the body,
susceptible of stimulation by certain methods, does the far-reaching change in the state of consciousness envisaged by Yoga become
possible. There is another unalterable condition. The nervous
system of the initiate must already have attained a certain degree
of preparedness, through heredity and a right mode of life, before
the manipulation or even the activity of the contrivance can be
effective enough to bear the desired fruit. It is because of the
formidable and unpredictable nature of the enterprise that the
ancients have likened the mysterious *kundalini,* the key to this
mechanism and power center, to a coiled serpent lying asleep on
the Manda, a triangular space with its apex downwards located
in the region bordering the lower end of the spinal column. Although there is some variation in the accounts of different authors
about the location of Kanda, the seat of *kundalini,* all are agreed

that the region lies somewhere between the perineum and the navel. The location of the *muladhara* and the other *cakras* is also meticulously described, though there are slight variations in these accounts also. These facts also clearly show that *kundalini*, being localized in space, must be a physiological contrivance, and, therefore, the channel or *nadis* through which it operates must also have a physical existence. How the whole region associated with *kanda* becomes active on the awakening of the serpent power, radiating energy to all the vital organs and centers, to effect rejuvenation of the body and elevation of mind will be described in another place in this volume.

In the light of these facts it would be a mistake to suppose that because the accounts of *nadis* do not exactly tally with our present chart of the nervous system, and because the alleged existence of the lotuses and other objects at the *cakras* has no substance in reality, the allusions made to them in the Tantras and other manuals on Kundalini-Yoga do not refer to the nerves made of flesh but to hypothetical channels of life energy interpenetrating the human body. If such were the case, then instead of suggesting the arduous and even dangerous practice of *pranayama,* which directly affects both the autonomic and the central nervous system, combined with postures, *mudras* and *bandhas* that are unequivocally physical exercises, the ancient masters would have contented themselves with recommending purely mental exercises to stimulate channels that had no corporeal reality, and could, therefore, be approached only through the medium of the mind. That from prehistoric times complicated, laborious, and painful psychosomatic methods have been used provides unmistakable evidence that the mechanism to be stimulated has an objective and concrete reality. When the mechanism has a corporeal existence the effects of its stimulation must have the semblance of a discernible psychic or biological activity, like the activity of other organs in the body. That it is so will become progressively apparent in the succeeding chapters in this volume.

It is true that universal *prana* is a superphysical substance like mind, but it has a tangible organic medium by which it acts on living organisms through specific channels of activity, that is, the cerebro-spinal system. We know very well that the brain is the instrument for the expression of mind. The only way by which we can come in contact with the supersensible realm of mind is by tuning the brain to finer vibrations not perceptible in the ordinary way. Whatever the method used to achieve the object—whether meditation, *pranayama, mantra,* or prayer—in every case the organ stimulated or affected is the brain or some specific portions of it about which we are still in the dark. What effect the training or tuning has or what changes occur in the nerves or the gray and white matter we do not know, but of this we have no doubt: all our practices and techniques finally impinge on the brain. The same is true word for word in the case of excitation of *kundalini. Prana* acts on our body through the nerves and the brain. It is, therefore, necessary in order to reach *kundalini* to direct our efforts to the training and tuning of both of them, which is exactly what the ancient authorities prescribe for the aspirants. For the arousal of *kundalini,* and for her subsequent activity, the somatic channel of the cerebro-spinal system is as necessary as the cultivation and development of the brain is necessary for the better expression of thought. Uncritical acceptance of the existing accounts, instead of elucidating, has made the subject more obscure and complicated and resulted in lending currency to false and misleading notions about this mighty power. The extent to which even the learned have been carried away by the cryptographic descriptions and cabalistic signs and diagrams is surprising. The common man has thus imbibed entirely erroneous ideas about this force, treating it as a supernatural power which, when propitiated or evoked with Yoga practices, puts an Aladdin's lamp into the hands of the fortunate Sadhaka to do with it as he likes.

Viewed apart from this huge and misleading mass of *cakras,* lotuses, shaktis, serpents, *mantras,* and other mythical creations of the human mind and interpreted in the light of modern knowledge, all that has a semblance of plausibility, and which we can accept subject to investigation, is the rather startling fact that the human body in the region close to the base of the spine has a reservoir of vital energy which, when activized with certain tried methods, leads to amazing changes in the human level of cognition, making the brain responsive to higher states of existence or to other dimensions of consciousness. This is a most extraordinary experience that has left its mark on history almost every time it became the destiny of the one who almost invariably blossomed into a prophet or an illumined sage. And this is not all. For the expression of a transcendent state of Consciousness a highly developed body, a superior nervous system and brain are the prerequisites demanded by nature to effect the transformation. The promises held out in the ancient texts about health and longevity are, therefore, to some extent, rooted in fact. Supernormal psychic gifts, such as prophecy and clairvoyance, as well as the power of fascination and magnetic appeal, also become available to the successful initiates within certain limits. This in a nutshell is the message of the Tantras and all the ancient treatises dealing with *kundalini*. In fact, as has been already explained, this is the aim and object of every form of Yoga, and every religious discipline. For the ultimate target of every occult or religious practice is to bring the mind in tune with Cosmic Consciousness or the Infinite Universe of Life, hidden from the normal mind. Supernormal psychic gifts, enhanced intellectual caliber, and literary talents invariably attend the crowning stages of the metamorphoses brought about.

The region contiguous to the base of the spine is lined with thick clusters of nerves and also forms a junction of a large number of arteries and veins. The nerves lining it come from both the central and the sympathetic nervous systems. This central area of the body forms the seat of the reproductive system in both men and women. There can be no denying the fact that human life, in its initial stages, is generated by this region and that from it arises the sexual impulse which has a most powerful effect on the brain. It is the seat of mystery and romance, of the yet unfathomed potentialities of life, of creativity as also of mental twists and obsessions of which psychology has only now begun to explore the depths. This part of the human anatomy has been an object of ceaseless speculation from the remotest epochs. It is often the first portion of the body to excite the curiosity of a child. It has been designed by Heaven, for reasons best known to it, to discharge, besides its normal function of procreation, the still nobler purpose of evolution, in conjunction with a specific center in the brain and a host of nerves, employed to extract the Elixir of Life from all parts of the body for transmission to it through a narrow duct in the spinal cord. This upward flow of the nerve energy, partly used for reproduction (*Urdhava-retas* in Sanskrit), forms the basis of Kundalini-Yoga. In fact, it is the ultimate aim of every form of Yoga, practiced for the attainment of transcendent states of consciousness. How the Elixir is transformed into a more powerful nerve current, which nerves are involved in this operation, what region of the brain is most affected, and how the transformation of consciousness takes place are questions which, to answer, would need the devoted labor of countless savants in times to come for a thorough exploration of what is one of the most momentous secrets of nature, underlying religion and every form of religious discipline, including Yoga. If we accept as true even a tithe of what the ancient masters claim for Kundalini-Yoga—superconsciousness, psychic powers, longevity, radiant health, genius, and a host of other gifts and talents —this points to a hidden source of energy and strength in the body, so marvelous, so potent, and so precious for the peace and happiness of mankind that no price paid for it and no sacrifice made to acquire the secret would be too great.

4

Yoga, True and False

According to some authorities on Yoga, one very essential qualification that should be present in an aspirant is *viveka* (discrimination). The person must be able to make up his mind as to
what is of real worth or of a permanent nature and what is un-
substantial and transitory. How necessary *viveka* is on the path of
liberation is expressed by Sankaracarya in Viveka-Cudamani (147)
in these words: "This bondage can be destroyed neither by
weapons nor by wind, nor by fire, nor millions of acts (enjoined
by scriptures): by nothing except the powerful sword of knowledge that comes of discrimination (*viveka*), sharpened by the grace
of the Lord." It is easy to see that as long as the aspirant has not
a correct sense of values and does not possess, in ample measure,
the faculty to determine what is really beneficial for him and
what is not, there is no possibility of his success in a difficult
enterprise like Yoga. *Viveka* is thus the very foundation stone
on which the subsequent efforts of an earnest seeker come to rest
for the simple reason that he himself has to make the choice of
the goal and the path he would like to pursue to reach it. Study
of books and scriptures or the advice of scholars and teachers can
only help to bring to his mind a whole bag, full of different goals
and different paths designed to reach them, advocated by different

authorities, each of them as learned, as pious, and as convincing as the other. But the choosing has to be done by the seeker alone, according to his own ability and his own power of discrimination, irrespective of what is suggested by others. It is here that the crux of the endeavor lies, for all the future harvest of his efforts depends on his choice.

In the search for a career, in the selection of a partner, or when embarking on a hazardous worldly enterprise do we not think deeply and debate within ourselves for days and weeks, even after consulting our friends and well-wishers, before making the final decision in the light of what appears to us most appropriate under the circumstances? What then should be our attitude when we try to reach God, the Author of Creation, or when we strive to gain entry to higher planes of consciousness which, as long as we have not found access to them, are deeper than the deepest bed of an ocean and farther than the farthest object on earth? If we have a genuine urge for this quest, should we not then wholeheartedly devote ourselves first to a deep study of the literature on this subject, especially to a study of the lives and utterances of those who are reported to have achieved the goal, to find out what kind of men they were, what obstacles beset them on the path, and what the reward was for their efforts, sacrifices, and sufferings at the end? This study, combined with a study of a few scriptures, as for instance the Bible, Quran, Bhagavad-Gita, Dhammapada, or any other Buddhist testament, will probably be enough to develop sufficient insight in an earnest seeker to enable him to determine the nature of the goal he should set before him and what he might expect at the end if his sincere efforts bear any fruit. If the approach to Yoga is made in this way, after weighing all the pros and cons, the conceptions about this science, in the minds of most people in both the East and West will undergo a radical transformation leading to a more healthy and sober view about this holy enterprise. It will then cease to have magical properties with which people invest it, and emerge as an objective reality with its full share of hazards, difficulties, disappointments and distractions, as any other enterprise undertaken by man.

The rarity of a successful consummation in Yoga is mainly due to the fact that most of those who embark on it have often no clearcut picture of the desired goal, how they themselves should be equipped for it, or what they should expect on the way. They usually accept the versions of the teachers whom they approach for guidance and who are often themselves unaware of the real goal and the path. They proceed to sit in the postures and to perform the other exercises as instructed by such teachers. In this way they bring down to the level of a mechanical, physical, or mental drill a system of discipline that is designed, in its true form, to reach down to the deepest levels of the human mind in order to effect radical changes in the whole psychological makeup of an individual. Commenting on the qualifications needed in a seeker for enlightenment, Updésa-Sāhasri writes: "This is always to be taught to one who is of tranquil mind, who has subjugated his senses, who is free from faults (of character), obedient, endowed with virtues, always submissive (to the teacher), and who is constantly eager for liberation."

Discrimination and dispassion are two of the most essential attributes needed in a Sadhaka, and every Indian scripture has accorded the highest priority to them. "But he (that master of the chariot, i.e., body)," says the Katha-Upanishad (1.3.7), "does not attain that goal, who being associated with a nondiscriminating intellect and an uncontrolled mind, is ever impure. He attains only worldly existence (involving birth and death)." During the probationary period, spent by the disciples with their teachers in India in ancient times, the latter had full occasion to frame their opinion about the merits of each disciple in the light of the injunctions contained in the sacred texts. This is clear from several passages in the Upanishads, as for instance Mundaka-Upanishad (1. 13): "To that pupil who has approached him with due courtesy, whose mind has become perfectly calm and who has control over his senses, the wise teacher should truly impart that knowledge of *Brahman* by which one realizes the Being, imperishable and real."

The Bhagavad-Gita repeatedly draws attention to the mental qualifications of the aspirants and time after time emphasizes the fact that without the basic virtues of detachment, self-mastery, devotion, faith and intellectual discrimination, success in the search for liberation is not possible. Self-control has to be acquired first before the actual practice of Yoga is started, "Pledged to the vow of continence, fearless, keeping himself perfectly calm and with the mind thoroughly brought under control and fixed on Me" says Krishna to Arjuna (iv. 14), "the vigilant Yogi should sit absorbed in Me." Again in vi. 36, He says: "Yoga is difficult of achievement for one whose mind is not subdued, but it can be easily attained with practice by him who with his mind under control ceaselessly strives for it; such is my belief." These citations make it abundantly clear, without the least trace of ambiguity, that a finely adjusted intellect, able to guide the Sadhaka in choosing his goal and his way of life and conduct is an indispensable prerequisite for the experience of Yoga. As at present Yoga is more or less an individual effort, with a great diversity in methods and innumerable exponents, each loud in the praise of his own method, the selection of a teacher needs the same fine exercise of the intellect as in all other matters. If this selection is not made with proper care there is every possibility of a failure even in the case of one who, after deep study and thought, has made the choice of the goal and the path which he would like to take.

This brings us to the very heart of the problem we wish to discuss. Since the time the various kinds of disciplines used in Yoga were first practiced or prescribed, a great transformation has occurred in the way of living, mode of thinking and social environment of people. The basic qualifications demanded for Yoga need a mode of life and certain attributes of mind, as for instance renunciation, self-denial and devotion, which are incompatible with the requirements of the present highly competitive and fast-moving age. The more sophisticated teachers, therefore, instead of advising their disciples to cultivate these essential attributes, and to adopt a concordant mode of life, make futile attempts to adapt the ancient teaching to the present highly artificial and competitive social order, often with disastrous consequences. The scope of this volume does not permit us to pursue this issue in detail. It is sufficient to point out here that there is gradually occurring a growing dissonance between the fundamental concept and practice of Yoga, as it was taught at the height of its spiritual practice in India in the past, and as it is now presented to the world. The impact of this calculated distortion has been especially harmful in the West for the reason that the seekers, having often no grounding in the scriptural lore of India, lack the necessary insight to differentiate between what the revealed texts prescribe and what the modern exponents try to inculcate.

From very early times there have been three classes of religious teachers and those dealing with the occult among whom it is necessary to distinguish in order to avoid waste of effort and disillusionment. One of the classes consists of those deeply versed in the sacred lore who have made themselves fully conversant with the details of various esoteric systems and religious disciplines, even practiced them, and who possess the ability to impress others with their knowledge and discourse. The second class comprises those who have diligently practiced the disciplines, possess or cultivate needed virtues, and who, as a result of long, ceaseless effort, attain a tranquil state of mind, have visionary experiences and develop, or are naturally gifted with, psychic powers, such as mind-reading, clairvoyance, etc., which they exhibit on occasions to instill respect in their followers. The third class, extremely limited and rare, consists of those who either as the result of a short or a long course of discipline, combined with lofty mental traits, an austere mode of life and exceeding benevolence of disposition, or as a natural endowment, attain the beatific state through psychic gifts, flashes of illumination and inspiration, and remain more in rapport with an entrancing inner rather than outer world. All systems of Yoga are designed to produce the mental state prevailing in the third category, which, because of the numerous factors involved and the radical nature of the transformation to be effected, becomes fruitful only in a few cases out of thousands who apply themselves to it.

The other two categories work with the light borrowed from the third, just named, which consists of a genuinely illumined class of men. The reason why they sometimes come to the fore-front is because the phenomenon of true spiritual efflorescence is extremely rare. "Out of thousands of men," says the Bhagavad-Gita (vii. 6) "hardly one strives for perfection and out of thousands of such seekers hardly one in reality attains to Me (Krishna as the Universal Self)." How difficult is the path for which enlightened teachers of the highest caliber are needed is described by Katha-Upanishad (1.3.14) in these words: "Arise, awake, and learn by approaching the Excellent Ones. The Wise describe that Path to be as impassable as a razor's edge, which when sharpened is difficult to tread on." Because of the fact that human beings, in general, are at different stages of development, both intellectual and moral, as they stand on different steps of the ladder of evolution, and have different tendencies and appetites, they have different ideas about perfection and the Ultimate as well, and are motivated by different aims in the quest for spiritual experience. Some seek worldly success and fulfillment of carnal desires with the aid of the magical gifts they hope to gain by this means. Others hanker after position and power and strive for the development of a magnetic personality, able to command the obedience of sundry people with the occult influences they will be able to radiate. Yet others are hungry for psychic gifts and supernormal faculties, clairvoyance, levitation and the like, and there are others who desire health, longevity, and a peaceful frame of mind under all circumstances. Few, indeed, there are who have actual knowledge of the real goal of Yoga and who long for the supreme experience, subordinating every other consideration and directing every other effort to this lofty aim.

Magic has been an ingredient of religion from the earliest times. In fact, in the "primitive" stages religion is indistinguishable from magic so much so that some scholars, among them J. G. Frazer, trace the origin of the former to it. Magic was much in evidence in India during the Vedic period and echoes of it are found in the Upanishads also. Thus in Brhadarnyaka a magical remedy is suggested to an injured husband (6.4.12) in this way: "Now if a man's wife has a lover and he wishes to hurt him, he should feed the fire in an unbaked earthen vessel, spread tips of reed inversely (to the usual way) and offer these inversely placed tips of reed, smeared with ghee (clarified butter), in the fire, uttering the following Mantras: 'Thou has offered in my burning fire thy *prana* and *apana,* I take them away, etc.' . . . 'Thou hast offered in my burning fire thy sons and cattle, I take them away, etc.' . . . " Patanjali has devoted the third book of his Yoga-Sutras to the enumeration of the supernormal gifts and miraculous powers attainable through the practice of Yoga. The Tantras and books on Hatha-Yoga are filled with magical rites, spells, charms and exercises for the attainment of fabulous powers and supernatural gifts. These excursions into the realm of magic and the miraculous, even on the part of great adepts of Yoga, have a profound relevance to human nature, since a large proportion of humanity has an innate propensity for the miraculous and the supernatural. In many cases this propensity is so strong that no amount of argument or dissuasion, and even no amount of proof to the contrary, can convince them that the domain of the supernatural is still shrouded in the darkness of doubt and suspicion, sometimes even trickery and fraud, and that demonstration of miraculous or magical powers by a person has seldom, if ever, been beyond dispute. In any case, it has never brought to him or to those who were benefited any lasting credit or good.

Accepting human nature as it is, the teachers of the two lower categories adapt their teaching to suit the predispositions of those whom they teach. The desire for supernatural adventure and the acquisition of miraculous powers, the subconscious longing in the heart of many people who take to Yoga and other occult practices, find a response in countless books, published in these days, which provide them liberally with many varieties of brightly colored and highly embellished foods, suited to their tastes. The old Tantric and Yoga texts of India and Tibet provide the raw material from which these appetizing dishes are cooked. The outcome has been that cheap and dangerous methods are taught to the unwary, and Yoga, brought down from its high pedestal, has been made a salable commodity which anyone can purchase for a price. Hypnotism, suggestion, drugs, magic, legerdemain, Mantras, and every other device known to man to excite curiosity for and to stimulate interest in the miraculous and the occult are all freely used by those who trade in the supernatural. The discriminating power of a balanced intellect, considered indispensable by the ancient masters for the right choice of the teacher and the path adopted, has been replaced by what is the most powerful incentive in this age: the possibility of gain. The aspirants seldom suspect that when a Guru breathes a Mantra into their ear and instructs them in meditation in a certain way, with the injunction that they should practice it daily in such-and-such a manner to gain such-and-such results is, without their knowledge, planting a suggestion deep into their subconscious and dealing with them in the same way as some mental healers and psychiatrists deal with the crowds of patients who throng their clinics or gather round them for treatment. The seekers after Yoga and the occult who, instead of counting on their own efforts, guided of course by a preceptor, display a weak mental attitude of utter dependence on the teacher for their spiritual regeneration, show evidence of lack of character and an unhealthy thirst for the Divine. Those who believe that they can attain to higher states of consciousness in this way, or by adopting any novel or easy method, deceive themselves and indirectly tend to cast a shadow of doubt and disrepute on this ancient science.

Hypnotism and suggestion have played a powerful role in all religious and occult practices from early times. The magical rites of the primitives and the occultists of Egypt, Chaldea, Greece, and other old civilizations made use of them in ample measure. The disciplines of Yoga contain a strong element of autohypnotism and suggestion in them. The attainment of a state of transcendent consciousness, which crowned the labors of most of the famous mystics, sages, and Yoga saints of the past, is a unique phenomenon, attended by certain well-marked attributes that can be objectively verified. In other cases, where the practitioners of spiritual disciplines, including Yoga, perceive visions, have supernatural visitations, or believe they have attained a state of mental calm, without developing the other talents which will be discussed in another chapter of this volume, and without experiencing a noteworthy change in their whole personality, are not infrequently experiencing the effects of autosuggestion, or the suggestion of an instructor that has gone home into the subconscious. Commenting on this possibility in the cases of conversion in his *Varieties of Religious Experience**, William James writes: "Similar occurrences abound, some with and some without luminous visions, all with a sense of astonished happiness, and of being wrought on by a higher control. If, abstracting altogether from the question of their value for the future spiritual life of the individual, we take them on the psychological side exclusively, so many peculiarities in them remind us of what we find outside of conversion that we are tempted to class them along with other automatisms, and to suspect that what makes the difference between a sudden and a gradual convert is not necessarily the presence of divine miracle in the case of one and of something less divine in that of the other, but rather a simple psychological peculiarity, the fact, namely, that in the recipient of the more instantaneous grace we have one of those subjects who are in possession of a large region in which mental work can go on subliminally, and from which invasive experiences, abruptly upsetting the equilibrium of the primary consciousness, can come."

It is undeniable that some cases of Yoga end merely in auto-

* Longmans, Green, New York, 1903.

hypnosis by causing the same condition of the brain as is deliberately induced by hypnotists in their subjects. Since some people are much more responsive to the hypnotic influence than others, it follows that the same rule must be true in respect of autohypnosis also, and that the more susceptible individuals succeed in inducing the condition in themselves more easily than others. Regular practice in a secluded place, a steady unmoving posture that can persist even when the mind passes into a sleeplike state, rhythmic breathing with soporific resonance proceeding from the monotonous utterance of specially selected words, fixity of attention or vacuity of thought create the passive or fatigued condition of the mind, favorable to the hypnotic trance. The idea already existing or inculcated about the Deity or the Superconscious state, acting as a suggestion, and using the now vivid imagination of the self-hypnotized Yoga practitioner, can create a hallucinatory appearance corresponding to it which has all the semblance of reality for him in the same way as a picture, evoked by the suggestion of a hypnotist, has for the moment a real existence for his subject. The vision is naturally accompanied by a state of happiness at the fulfillment of an earnest desire, which is reflected on the countenance of the Yogi.

Many of the secret rites and hidden practices, prescribed by esoteric systems and occult creeds as well as many exercises of Yoga, are but effective methods of self-hypnosis in disguise. They cause the practitioner to fall into a state of mental passivity leading to trance. The daily repetition of the experience tends to fortify belief in the reality of the vision and to create an assurance that the practitioner has found what he had striven for. This assurance has a powerful effect in creating self-confidence in him and in influencing his followers and disciples. Once the ability to induce hypnosis in himself has been gained by a Sadhaka, the next step of exhibition of psychic talents becomes possible soon afterward in a certain proportion of successful initiates. They may succeed in awakening extracerebral memories relating to the past or in exhibiting clairvoyance, prevision or other supernormal gifts.

As these extrasensory developments do not occur in all successful cases of self-hypnosis but only in a few, in the manner of hypnotized subjects, it is obvious that the condition supervenes only in such cases where a tendency already exists in the brain in a dormant form and only needs some stimulus to stir it and bring it out.

This class of Yogis and occultists, though much more numerous than the true Yoga saints and mystics, and existing from prehistoric times, has made no impact on mankind, though in their own circumscribed environment men of this category shine brilliantly for a while. The reason for this is simple. They do not possess the ever-shining light of genius nor the dynamic power of the soul to shed a luster that could survive beyond the narrow span of their lives. Apart from the fact that they can induce the condition in themselves, and on that account possess confidence in their own ability to cause the phenomena, Yogis of this class are in other respects no better than hypnotized subjects or professional sensitives and mediums, whose demonstrations are witnessed by thousands every year. It is a mistake to suppose that they can produce these extraordinary phenomena at will and mold the occult forces of nature according to their choice. If it were so and they did possess the power of command over these forces, they could dispel the doubts of the multitudes with but one conclusive supernatural demonstration before the skeptics, whose number is alarmingly on the increase, and with but one bodily flight in the air, while the cameras are recording and thousands of eyes witnessing the feat, revive belief in the occult for at least many centuries to come. But no such demonstration has ever been ventured, nor is likely to be ventured for a long time to come. It can be readily admitted that there are hidden powers and occult forces in nature about which modern scholars are still in the dark. But, as in the case of material energies, they too must be governed by rigid and uniform laws. They await the time when man can make lawful use of them with full understanding of their nature and possibilities. Till that day the erratic exhibitions, witnessed in mediums and others, can only be treated as freakish occurrences, which, in the course of time, with study and investigation, may lead to a better understanding of their origin and the purpose they can serve.

The material phenomena, attributed to prophets, mystics and Yogis, though counterfeited to some extent by mediums and sensitives in their seance chambers during recent times, have never been conclusively demonstrated. They have never even been unequivocally proved in the past, because if this had been done it would have shut, once and for all, the mouths of the skeptics and unbelievers who at no time in history ceased to cast doubts on the Divine and the supernatural. To what extent the skeptical attitude was in evidence in the past is also amply illustrated in the dialogue of the Buddha in which he explicitly states that the exhibition of supernatural feats on the part of one on a spiritual path instead of enhancing his reputation is more likely to result in his classification as a mountebank and trickster. It is said that when informed by a disciple that a certain monk had flown up to the top of a high pole, and thence circled the town three times, to win a sandalwood bowl, which a rich merchant had placed on the top of the pole with the proclamation that one who could take it from there would possess it, Buddha ordered the bowl to be broken into pieces and distributed.

Leaving aside the psychics and mediums, some of whose exhibitions, especially of the material kind, lack coherence and consistency and need further investigation for their verification after eliminating every possibility of fraud and trickery, we have now only two classes of men to deal with. One class is the prophets, Yoga saints and mystics, and the other class those Yogis and holy men, who as a result of autosuggestion or self-hypnosis develop a conviction that they have attained a state of illumination and that the visions and appearances they perceive in trance or semitrance states, are real manifestations of the Divine and not mere figments of their own voluntarily excited imaginations. These two classes have been mentioned to demonstrate the main compartments into which Yogis and those who strive for God-realization can be roughly divided.

Dehydration and deprivation of water for some time in a desert, the rarity of air on a high mountain peak, prolonged starvation or numbness by exposure to extreme cold can cause hallucinations in which the victim ceases to experience the agony which torments him. From this analogy it is safe to infer that prolonged fasting, extreme austerity, and self-mortification as well as too little sleep, a state of excessive preoccupation with the supernatural and the numinous, in utter silence and solitude, cannot but predispose the mind toward obsessions and delusions that may even take the form of hallucinatory manifestations. The morbid effects of unnatural modes of life and repression of natural tendencies are now too well known to require mention. In the light of this knowledge it should not be difficult to understand the state of mind of an anchorite, whose life is a bundle of inhibitions, fastings, self-denials, and mortifications of the flesh with excessive attention given to the unseen and the unknowable. Is it then to be wondered that after a time the mind loses its grip on reality and lives in a world of fantasies and dreams?

It is a fact well known to hypnotists that, after a subject has been once subjected to a hypnotic trance, it becomes much easier on subsequent occasions to induce the sleep by means of a single gesture, a word of command, a look, or a suggestion. In rare cases, where the subject is responsive to telepathy, even a mental command from a distance is sometimes sufficient to bring about the hypnosis. This also holds true in the case of autohypnosis. Once a Sadhaka succeeds in inducing in himself the hypnotic trance, it becomes easier for him on subsequent attempts to induce this alluring state when the ideas present in his mind materialize in self-caused visions of extraordinary vividness, appearing much more real and substantial than the most vivid experiences in dreams. No wonder then that some of them exude an atmosphere of such poise and calm, and are so confident of the reality of their own visionary experiences that they often exercise a powerful effect on those who sit in their company contrasting their serene bearing with the agitated minds of other people.

Those of them who gain access to the deeper regions of the mind and succeed in developing dormant psychic faculties command even greater homage and excite greater wonder among the people who witness these extraordinary feats. Since most of us are not yet fully informed about the identity of the factors that work in a hypnotized subject and a self-hypnotizing Yogi causing the trance and the psychic phenomena, we fail to recognize the similarity between the two. Although this form of Yoga has its benefits it has its disadvantages as well. The initiate, it is true, can voluntarily dive into the depths of his subconscious, but that only means descending into a dream-state, not as one does in sleep, but with deliberation plunging into a hallucinatory condition, transported to a world of being where thoughts take on a visionary aspect and fancies assume vivid appearances somewhat akin to the illusory states induced by drugs. At best it can only signify volitional excursions into the dream territory, often with some therapeutic results, but nothing more. There is at present a general ignorance about the fact that the practice of Yoga, or for that matter of any form of religious discipline, can lead to two fundamentally different mental states. One is brought about by autohypnosis, creating a hallucinatory inner world of visions, with or without psychic powers. The other is a state of transformed consciousness, leading to glorious supersensory planes of being, attended always by genius and psychic powers in one form or another characteristic of all great seers, prophets, mystics, and Yogis of the past.

The following extract from Aldous Huxley's work, *Heaven and Hell,** can help to illustrate our meaning: "Some people never consciously discover their antipodes. Others make an occasional landing. Yet others (but they are few) find it easy to go and come as they please. For the naturalist of the mind, the collector of psychological specimens, the primary need is some safe, easy and

* Harper & Row, New York, 1956.

reliable method of transporting himself and others from the old world to the new, from the continent of the familiar cows and horses to the continent of the wallaby and the platypus. . . . Two such methods exist. Neither of them is perfect; but both are sufficiently reliable, sufficiently easy and sufficiently safe to justify their employment by those who know what they are doing. In the first case, the soul is transported to its far-off destination by the aid of a chemical—either mescalin or lysergic acid. In the second case, the vehicle is psychological in nature, and the passage to the mind's antipodes is accomplished by hypnosis. The two vehicles carry the consciousness to the same region; but the drug has the longer range and takes its passengers further into the terra incognita." The passages denote a poor concept of the Ineffable or rather the very antithesis of the true mystical state. What Huxley is describing are visionary or rather hallucinatory excursions into below-the-surface levels of the mind while the unitive state is a flight to regions beyond the farthest reach of submerged states.

How and why hypnosis produces its observed effects Huxley, or for that matter psychologists, are not able to explain. "All that is necessary, in this context," Huxley says, "is to record the fact that some hypnotic subjects are transported, in the trance state, to a region in the mind's antipodes, where they find the equivalent of marsupials—strange psychological creatures leading an autonomous existence according to the law of their own being."* About the physiological effect of mescalin, Huxley offers the explanation that probably it interferes with the enzyme system that regulates cerebral functioning and by so doing lowers the efficiency of the brain as an instrument for focusing the mind on the problems of life. "This lowering of the biological efficiency of the brain seems to permit," he says, "the entry into consciousness of certain classes of mental events, which are normally excluded, because they possess no survival value. Similar intrusions of biologically useless, but aesthetically and sometimes spiritually valuable, material may occur as the result of illness or fatigue; or they may be

* *Ibid.*

induced by fasting, or a period of confinement in a place of darkness and complete silence." At another place he adds: "Milarepa,
in his Himalayan cavern, and the anchorites of the Thebaid followed essentially the same procedure and got essentially the same
results. A thousand pictures of the Temptations of St. Anthony
bear witness to the effectiveness of restricted diet and restricted environment. Asceticism, it is evident, has a double motivation. If
men and women torment their bodies, it is not only because they
hope in this way to atone for past sins and avoid future punish-
ments, it is because they long to visit the mind's antipodes and do
some visionary sightseeing. Empirically and from the reports of
other ascetics, they know that fasting and a restricted environment
will transport them where they long to go,"

These passages reveal an intellectual confusion, common among
some scholars and people in general, about the sublime experience
of the genuine mystical state. This confusion has prevailed from
time immemorial, with the result that the rigid ascetic who starved
himself or employed other methods of self-mortification to induce
a hallucinatory state of mind, by causing alterations in the physiological balance of the body, has often been mistakenly bracketed
with the true mystic or the illumined sage. In actual fact the two
conditions are poles apart. One denotes a decline and the other a
high degree of enhancement of the mental faculties. This is a
point of paramount importance to be kept in mind in determining the value of Yoga or any other healthy form of spiritual discipline. The vision of God or contact with Cosmic Consciousness
to be genuine must signify a step forward and not a recession in
the mental condition of the seeker. The reason for some people
taking hallucinatory drugs or employing other methods to gain
visionary or illusory experiences springs from a misconception of
the value of genuine mystical phenomena. If the urge to realize
Divinity or have access to higher planes of being, which has been a
powerful influence in the life of man from earliest times, has as
its final aim the fantasmic states induced by hormone-derange-
ment, starvation, or drugs, it clearly points to an unwholesome

impulse at work in the human psyche which, under the guise of leading man to his Maker, draws him into a world of appearances and apparitions only slightly removed from the borderline of insanity.

Referring to the consciousness produced by intoxicants and anesthetics, especially by alcohol, William James says*: "The sway of alcohol over mankind is unquestionably due to its power to stimulate the mystical faculties of human nature, usually crushed to earth by the cold facts and dry criticisms of the sober hour. Sobriety diminishes, discriminates, and says no; drunkenness expands, unites and says yes. It is in fact the great exciter of the Yes function in man. It brings its votary from the chill periphery of things to the radiant core. It makes him for the moment one with truth. . . . The drunken Consciousness is one bit of the mystic Consciousness, and our total opinion of it must find its place in our opinion of that large whole." . . . "Nitrous oxide and ether," he continues, "especially nitrous oxide, when sufficiently diluted with water, stimulate the mystical consciousness in an extraordinary degree. Depth beyond depth of truth seems revealed to the inhaler. This truth fades out, however, or escapes, at the moment of coming to, and if any words remain over in which it seemed to clothe itself, they prove to be the veriest nonsense. Nevertheless, the sense of a profound meaning having been there persists, and I know more than one person who is persuaded that in the nitrous oxide trance we have a genuine metaphysical revelation."

The confusion is due to the fact that a standard, clearcut picture of what a true mystic experiences in the highest flights of ecstasy is not available anywhere. In the first place the condition is incommunicable and, second, its range of expression is so vast and there are such enormously varied accounts of it that it is extremely difficult to locate the boundary at which the spurious forms, induced by hallucinogens, etc., cease and the genuine oc-

* *Varieties of Religious Experience* by William James, Longmans, Green, New York, 1903.

currences begin. This issue will find clarification in another chapter of this volume. In India the genuine Yogis with a transformed consciousness usually met instant recognition throughout the past. The learned scholar, the miracle-worker, and the one prone to drugs also had their place among the holy men, but they were in the lower ranks. The Hindu scriptures are categorical in their emphasis on a regulated life and a disciplined mind for one practicing Yoga. The extremes of the type that lead to morbid states of the mind or to foods and drinks that cause unhealthy reactions in the body have to be eschewed. In fact, some of the caste restrictions about food arise from the scriptural injunctions that food, being the builder of *prana*, must be pure and wholesome.

That the mental condition induced by nitrous oxide is hallucinatory is obvious from the fact, mentioned by William James, that on emerging from the visionary state the words in which the truth witnessed in the trance condition clothes itself are found to be sheer nonsense. The return to normalcy from all the hallucinogens and intoxicants that cause a temporary inflation of personality is almost always followed by feelings of depression or lassitude. The aftereffects of genuine ecstasy are altogether different. The genuinely esctatic experience is revealed as if a heaven has been opened. The sublime nature of the vision, surpassing anything known or even imagined in the normal state, remains indelibly engraved on the memory, an unending source of inspiration and wonder which, even in the darkest hours of life, sustains the spirit with hope and cheer. Sometimes even one fleeting glimpse of the supreme state continues to shine in the depths of the heart as a beacon pointing to a glorious existence that does not belong to this daily world. St. Ignatius Loyola* has described one such experience that befell him in these words (He refers to himself in the third person): "As he was going to pay his devotions at the Church of St. Paul, about a mile out of the town of Manresa, and was sitting on the banks of the Cardenero, or as

* *Spiritual Exercises*, translated from the Spanish by Anthony Mottolo. Garden City, New York, 1964.

some say of the Rubricato, his mind was suddenly filled with a
new and strange illumination, so that in one moment, and without any sensible image or appearance, certain things pertaining to
the mysteries of the Faith, together with other truths of natural
science, were revealed to him, and this so abundantly and so
clearly, that he himself said, that if all the spiritual light which
his spirit had received from God up to the time when he was
more than sixty-two years old, could be collected into one, it
seemed to him that all this knowledge would not equal what was
at that moment conveyed to his soul."

The true prophets, mystics and Yoga saints constitute a class
of men including in its ranks the founders of all religions, as well
as several great systems of metaphysics and philosophy, initiators
of new lines of thought and conduct, adepts in the knowledge of
the occult and originators or reformers of all systems of religious
discipline and Yoga. Not one of them veiled his identity or hid
himself and the Light he came to diffuse in a far-away mountain
retreat, but, on the contrary, boldly fought the evils of his time
and valiantly stood against the tyranny and wrath not only of rep-
robate kings and chiefs but also of powerful heads of corrupt
religions and prevailing decadant creeds. These mystics proved an
asset to the country in which they were born.

Misconceptions about this subject in the minds of the common
people in this enlightened age are due to the fact that the modern
world, though immensely rich in physical science, is deplorably
lacking in knowledge of the occult and the sublime. The inherent
tendency in the human mind to associate mystery and wonder with
the Divine, for which there is a rational ground deprived of the
proper nourishment, is driven to feed itself voraciously on a
fictitious other-world, on the hair-raising tales of ghosts and
haunted houses, on incredible stories of hypothetical miracle-
working supermen and hierarchic Methuselahs living in inaccessible regions, which has done, and is doing, great harm by diverting
the attention of the true seekers from the understanding of a
mighty law of nature by which man can raise himself to a sub-

lime state in a most rational way as natural and as practical as the birth and development of a child. This unwholesome diet has caused serious harm in several directions. On the one hand, it aggravates the mental condition and makes the appetite even more morbid and, on the other, draws the attention from the genuine ideals and diverts it toward persons or concepts of the occult and the Divine that are either fictitious and have no relation to reality or are not at all fit to form the models worthy of emulation by mankind.

Approached in a sane way the realm of the occult and the supernatural will also be found to be crowded with the fictitious and the spurious, as in any worldly realm. Those who do so will find that, barring the experience of those prophets, mystics and Yoga sages, whose names are household words in the countries to which they belong, all the rest they have heard about such as the imaginary adepts and wonder-workers do not possess the seal of attestation either of those who were a witness to their extraordinary lives, or of the monuments they left behind to show that they were men or women of flesh and blood. The utmost they will discover of the occult, in the objective world, well attested and confirmed, will be the erratic and unpredictable phenomena produced by sensitives, mediums, hypnotized subjects, or some self-hypnotizing Yogis, but beyond that, nothing. If they try to bring before their minds the image of the most outstanding seer or Yogi they have ever heard of, out of the known and well-attested cases, they will find that he is something quite different from what they themselves would wish to be. They will also find that almost all the illuminati, about whom they have heard, had lives of suffering, of intense longing for the Divine, sometimes almost to the point of madness, of utter simplicity and self-denial, of detachment from the world and renunciation of its pleasures, of selfless service, often in the face of colossal odds and insurmountable difficulties, of complete immersion in the love of the Deity and entire absorption in the inner universe. They can easily gather from this that success in the quest, if ever attained, would add their names to the same category, and fill their minds with the same fires of passion, renunciation, love of the Divine, and service for humanity that characterized the illuminati.

It is well known that in both medieval and ancient times the men and women, who delved into the occult in order to become sorcerers, magicians, necromancers, wizards, or witches were never publicly applauded. They were forced to practice in secret, to form esoteric circles and brotherhoods, and to perform their weird rites far from the eyes of common men, in eerie spots and in the shades of night. Modern man, deceived by the fictitious accounts he has read, and filled with the glamorous images of hypothetical Master Yogis, is too often led to believe that a few years practice with certain secret methods would raise him to the same level, able to achieve impossible deeds with the power gained over the forces of nature, to conquer disease, to win domination over men, to know the deeper secrets of life, and to live in utter peace and bliss under all circumstances. How many men succeed in achieving these objectives can be gauged from the fact that in recent years out of the millions, who undertook the practice of Yoga, not one has claimed that he has gained even a fraction of the powers claimed for it or for other forms of esoteric discipline by the over-enthusiastic protagonists of these systems. Leaving miraculous powers aside, how many have plainly or implicitly made the assertion that they, in their person, have attained the transcendent state of Consciousness claimed for Yoga, and backed their assertions by a frank self-revelation in the same way as has been done by several well-known Christian mystics, Sufis, and Yoga saints in the past with a candor and sincerity that has made their works immortal? If there is none or only one or two, it clearly points to the fact that the present way of approach to Yoga holds little promise of success for the legions who undertake it in these days.

By miraculous powers we mean the type of supernatural talents which legendary Yogis like Gorajah Nath are said to have exercised, that is, the type of powers mentioned by Patanjali in his Yoga-Sutras under the term *siddhis* and which are repeated in almost all the books on Kundalini- and Hatha-Yoga. This does not refer to uncontrollable psychic gifts, which hundreds of mediums possess, but to the power of will developed to an extent where one can exercise the occult faculties, under all circumstances and in full view of people in broad day light, and can repeat the same performance at any time at his choice. The interruption of breathing, of the heart action, or of other functions of the body, including the flow of blood, are merely physical phenomena and do not fall in the category of occult powers, referred to here. Many of the present-day concepts about the supernatural and the occult are purely mythical. But the myth is so prevalent and so concordant with our wishful thinking that, despite every indication to the contrary and the fact that hundreds of thousands of disillusioned seekers bear testimony to the repeatedly proven hollowness of many of these beliefs, a large number of those interested in the occult still persist in the quest. They convince themselves that had such extraordinary achievements not been possible, then countless men would not have devoted their lives to this pursuit from time immemorial. Others console themselves with the thought that were there not a substratum of truth in such episodes all these stories of supermen could not have found currency or commanded such wide acceptance.

As has been explained, the Yogi whose image has been projected on the public mind, especially in the West, by some modern exponents of the occult, exists nowhere in the world. There is no Yogi who readily changes from the physical into the astral body, conveys his instructions by mental projection, heals with a touch, transmutes base metals into gold, transforms his disciples into adepts, or performs other similar miracles while leading a happy, unruffled life free from the cares of the world. At least history makes no mention of any such extraordinary spiritual prodigy or Yogi who in his own person rose above physical laws, performed miracles left and right, and lived a life of peace and happiness to the end. On the other hand, in all saints and mystics of the world we come across lives of spiritual storm and stress, of a raging passion for divine experience, of periods of intense joy interspersed with spells of extreme despair, of persecutions and martyrdom, of extreme poverty and want, of ravaging disease and premature deaths, or rigid austerities and self-mortification, of ridicule and calumny, of great trials and suffering and other vicissitudes, in many cases far more severe and trying than are often met with in ordinary lives.

Time and again the author of the Bhagavad-Gita gives an insight into the mental condition of the accomplished Yogi. The Herculean struggle for self-mastery, the extremely recalcitrant nature of the mind, the moderate, well-balanced life that must be led, the awful yet blissful nature of the supreme vision, the pitfalls in the path, the pattern of behavior to be followed, the mental attributes of the emancipated, the dangers of employing psychic powers, the sacrifices and surrenders to be made are all described at length. There are many people who after years of ceaseless efforts, sacrifice, and suffering find no change in their state of consciousness, and in the essential aspects of their personality continue to be the same as they were before. In their despair they either blame the teacher or the whole system which they followed or even question the justice of the divine Being toward whom all their devotion, sacrifice, and effort were directed. Why there should be such a reaction is based on the mistaken idea that all our spiritual endeavor is a means to please or propitiate the Lord and to seek His grace in order to cross over to the other shore. Is it not an anomaly that while, in the intellectual sphere, out of millions who devote their lives to the various sciences and arts and make colossal sacrifices to win distinction in them, only an extremely few rise to the stature of a Shakespeare, a Kalidasa, an Omar Khayyam or a Confucius. The rest reasonably attribute the rise to exceptional natural talent, based on some still unknown biological law. In the spiritual realm the seekers after God do not often take the same reasonable view and, instead of attributing their failure to a law of nature, assign other causes for it.

The true aim of Yoga is transformation of Consciousness, the creation of a heaven on earth. What lasting joy can supernormal talents or command over supernatural forces bring to a man whose inner being has not risen above the narrow, vacillating periphery of the human mind. What greater happiness can occult gifts, temporal power, or earthly riches confer on a man who, in perennial communion with the Universal Ocean of Life, has realized his own immortal nature, knows himself as one with the Eternal Fount of Cosmic Consciousness, in want of nothing and beyond the farthest reach of the contaminations of the earth: sorrow, decay and death. The other subsidiary achievements, supernormal gifts and powers of domination, after which many people strive, are but alluring pitfalls in the path. The object to be realized is the experience of the Self, beyond all price, beyond all thought and beyond everything the earth can offer. This is how Chandogya Upanishad (iii–14–2 & 3) has tried to depict this state:—"He, who is permeating the mind, who has Prana for his body, whose nature is consciousness . . . who possesses all the agreeable odours and all the pleasant tastes, who exists pervading all this, who is without speech (and other senses). . . . This my Atman residing in (the lotus of) the heart is greater than the earth, greater than the sky, greater than heaven, greater than all these worlds."

This idea is re-echoed by Lao Tze in his Tao-Te-Ching (85 and 89): "Of old these came to be in possession of the One; Heaven in virtue of the One is limpid; Earth in virtue of the One is settled; Gods in virtue of the One have their potencies; the valley in virtue of the One is full; the Myriad creatures in virtue of the One are alive; lords and princes in virtue of the One become leaders in the empire; it is the One that makes these what they are; . . . The Myriad creatures in the world are born from something, and Something from Nothing." The supreme experience of Yoga or other forms of religious discipline is unlike any other experience known to the mind. It is more real and more convincing, whether undergone in the trance state or in full wakefulness, than any objective experience undergone by anyone during the whole course of embodied life.

5

The Discipline of Yoga

As the various methods for the awakening of *kundalini,* described
in Hatha-Yoga manuals or prescribed in other ancient texts, are
already mentioned in detail in several modern books, it is not
necessary here to enter into a recapitulation of the techniques
already explained in other writings. A few words are, however,
necessary to bring out the fact that all the practices and exercises
described are of a type that one would expect of a system, designed for the excitation of a psychosomatic mechanism in the
body, intimately connected with the reproductive region at the
base of the spine and the cerebral hemispheres in the head. The
ancient writers on the subject have made no secret of this close
relationship between the two poles of the mechanism, and even the
purest and the most saintly of them have described the interaction
of the two in plain terms without any effort at ambiguity. In
assessing the value of the ancient techniques it is necessary to bear
in mind that they were designed at a time when knowledge of the
human body was extremely meager and recourse to supernatural
agencies and spiritual forces to account for the more obscure
functions of the organism which are not clearly defined in biological terms was very common. When once the processes responsible
for spiritual experience are rightly understood in the context of

biology, the development of new techniques and more improved methods will follow instantly as a matter of course.

Patanjali divides the whole process of Yoga into eight parts, or limbs. These are *yama* (restraint), *niyama* (discipline), *asana* (posture), *prana-yama* (control of breathing), *pratyahara* (control of senses), *dharana* (concentration), *dhyana* (unbroken contemplation), and *samadhi* (complete absorption). The Hatha-Yoga and Laya-Yoga have also the same eight divisions. There are minor differences in respect of the subdivisions of each part. The Yoga-Sutras specify five *yamas* and five *niyamas,* and the manuals of Hatha-Yoga ten of each. Briefly stated the *yamas* are avoidance of violence to living creatures, truth, absence of covetousness, forbearance, fortitude, kindness, simplicity, moderation in food, and purity of body and of mind. The *niyamas* are austerity, contentment, belief in scriptures, charity, worship, listening to holy texts, repugnance for wrongful action, adherence to scriptural ordinances, recitation of sacred formulas, and practice of religious observances.

Broadly speaking the ordinances grouped under the heads of *yama* and *niyama* are the rules of conduct and behavior to be observed by every aspirant to spiritual illumination. They are designed to inculcate the ideals of truth, piety, harmlessness, charity, self-control, and altruism without which no spiritual achievement is possible. In the Bhagavad-Gita the qualifications of one fit for the supreme experience have been repeatedly and variously defined.

There is no doubt that the most important contribution of religion to the progress of mankind has been morality. From the earliest times the ideas of forbidden and permissible, of sacred and profane, of clean and polluted, of pure and impure formed the raw material from which the subsequent towering edifices of morality and ethics were built. Both in primitive societies and in later civilized cultures the evolutionary impulse was at the bottom of the ethical tendency in the primary crude and subsequent elaborated forms.

If it is conceded that man has a spiritual goal to attain, and there is certainly no conflict of opinion about this point, at least among the various faiths of mankind, it follows that, in order to make this idea a reality, the spirit must gain more and more domination over the flesh and not be dominated by it, since that would be a step in the opposite direction toward carnality and bondage and not toward emancipation. This implies that rise in morality denotes a rise in the power of the spirit. From this the conclusion is obvious that any discipline or method designed to gain self-realization or God-consciousness must be oriented to raise the moral stature of the practitioner to a level where it can offer no hindrance in gaining self-mastery to the enlightened soul.

For this reason self-denial, control of the senses, detachment from the world, truth and right conduct form the necessary ingredients of every kind of Yoga and every school of religious discipline. As it is in the nature of men to go to the extreme, the scriptural injunctions and the spirit of the commandments have too often been distorted or highly exaggerated with the result that excessive forms of self-denial and detachment, instead of a healthy and judicious moderation, have been and are frequently practiced to forge even stronger bonds around the soul by causing obsessive and morbid states of the mind. The vast majority of the seers of the Upanishads were householders and lived healthy and meritorious normal lives to a mature age, when they entered the third stage and retired to the forests to strive for enlightenment. The successful termination of this effort led later to the fourth stage, or *ashrama,* when the now accomplished sage wandered as a homeless ascetic, welcomed and revered everywhere, to allay the doubts and answer the questions of those deeply interested in the mighty problems of life and death. One of the greatest of these sages, Yajnavalkya, discredits severe austerity and self-mortification as effective means for *Brahman*-realization. In the Mundaka Upanishad continence, truth, and performance of prescribed duties are considered to be sufficient measures for the attainment of higher consciousness. The Bhagavad-Gita strongly condemns excessive penance and self-mortification, preaching moderation, self-less action, devotion, truth, and righteousness as the most appropriate virtues of those who seek enlightenment.

Considering the arduous nature of the psycho-physiological discipline, and the long duration of mental exercises, it is but natural that certain postures of the body should have been chosen for the *asana* stage. Beyond this, *asanas* have no other significance in other forms of Yoga and, according to both Patanjali and the Gita, the Sadhaka himself has to make the choice of the way in which to seat himself, remaining steady and keeping the head, torso, and neck erect to avoid flexion of the spinal cord. In the Hatha-Yoga, however, in order to prepare the body for a sudden infusion of the life force as the result of a powerful awakening of the serpent power, *asanas* are also used to limber one up to a state of toughness and flexibility necessary for the proper functioning of the visceral organs. The statement in the Gheranda Samhita that there are 8,400,000 *asanas,* of which 1,600 are said to be excellent, is obviously an exaggeration, a specimen of the manner in which a simple fact is presented in an entirely incredible manner in some of the ancient texts, demanding a sane and critical approach on the part of the seeker. The number of *asanas* actually described in this work is only thirty-two. Hatha-Yoga Pradipaka describes fifteen *asanas* only.

Shiva Samhita mentions eighty-four postures and this number is usually accepted even now. There are Sadhus in India who can perform most of these *asanas* with alacrity for a small gift. They are as far away from Yoga as any body-training gymnast or acrobat is. It is as great a misnomer to call efficiency in the mere performance of a few difficult and striking *asanas* Yoga as it would be to designate a dextrous circus performer as a Yogi. The Yogic *asanas,* when employed merely for gaining suppleness and health of the body, are no better than other body-building exercises, and ought to be understood and labeled as such. The assertions made in Hatha-Yoga treatises that miraculous powers attend the proper performance of certain *asanas* are an obvious exaggeration, used as an inducement to the seekers for undertaking the disciplines. The two most convenient *asanas* for any kind of Yoga are the *padmasana* and the *siddhasana*. In the former the right foot is placed on the left thigh and the left foot on the right thigh, with the heels pressing against the pudenda, and the hands either placed in a similar manner, the right hand on the left thigh and vice versa, or simply each hand on the thigh of the same side. In the other *asana* one heel is pressed against the perineum and the other against the region of the genitals, with the hands on the thighs or one upon the other, palms upward, on the upper leg.

Every Sadhaka can select a convenient posture for himself out of the many enumerated in Yoga manuals, but for an earnest seeker, whose mind is set on *samadhi*, the posture should be one which he can maintain for hours without fatigue or cramp, and which keeps his head and trunk steady and unflexed. A few words are here necessary to explain the significance of the gruesome *asanas* peculiar to some schools of Tantric Yoga, in which the Sadhaka performs the practice in a cremation ground or seated on a skull or astride a corpse. The use of human skulls and bones in the performance of occult practices has been in vogue from very early times and prevailed in many places in one form or the other. In the mystery cults of Chaldea, Greece, and Egypt, revolting and fear-exciting ceremonies, as for instance the kissing of snakes, embracing a dead person's hand, infliction of wounds, and the shedding of blood, were held to instill a sense of respect and awe with regard to the mysterious ritual into which the candidate was initiated. In the light of these practices there is nothing new or surprising in the *mundasana* and *shavasana* of some Tantrics and the utter indifference to what they eat, not excluding even dung, of the Aghoris.

The six processes of body-cleaning are: (1) *Dhauti.* This is a method to clean the mouth, throat, stomach, and intestines by swallowing a long piece of wet cloth and then drawing it out. The other accessories to this process are drinking a copious draught of water and then expelling it through the mouth, contraction and expansion of the abdominal and intestinal muscles to eject wind, self-stimulated vomiting and muscular contractions, combined with pressure of the breath, to cause increase or decrease in the peristaltic movement of the entire digestive tract at will. (2) *Vasti*. This is a method by which a Yogi, sitting in a stream or pool up to the navel, can draw up water through the anus by means of suction applied with the action of breath and the intestinal muscles combined, and after cleaning the lower portion of the tract, eject it. (3) *Neti*. This means thorough cleansing of the nasal passages by the use of a thread. (4) *Lauliki*. This is achieved by the movement of the contracted abdominal muscles from side to side to ensure regular motion of the bowels and to maintain the suppleness of the waist. (5) *Trataka*. This is an exercise at concentration and strengthening the muscles of the eye by gazing fixedly at some object without winking. (6) *Kapalabhati*. This is a method for the removal of phlegm and mucus by means of breathing exercises or by drawing up water through the nose and ejecting it through the mouth and vice versa.

It is obvious that years of practice are required in order to gain proficiency in these exercises. What purpose could this difficult and even precarious system of body-cleansing fulfill in the attainment of a higher state of consciousness, is a question that can arise in the mind of any student of Hatha-Yoga. To take only one instance, the exercise of *trataka* in the hands of an ignorant Sadhaka can do great damage to the eyes. Sometimes this practice degenerates into gazing at the sun with disastrous results and loss of eyesight of the unfortunate seekers after Yoga. What unbending necessity could drive the experts to devise and practice such rough methods of internal cleanliness, especially of the stomach and the intestinal tract? As far as we know the only reason offered for these practices is that they are needed to correct the inequality of the three humors and to keep the body in a healthy condition. But why such drastic methods were undertaken when drugs to cause vomiting and even contrivances to clean the colon were available in India in ancient times is not clear. There can be only

two answers to the question: either these practices were undertaken for their wonder-exciting property, which appears hardly
plausible as more amazing performances, such as sleeping on a
bed of nails or standing on one leg or living atop a tree, were
possible with less labor and the chances of a greater yield, or there
is something inherent in this form of Yoga which makes proficiency in the methods of body-cleansing a necessary qualification
in a candidate for sublime spirituality, and for this reason years
were spent in gaining mastery over them.

According to the ancient treatises on Hatha-Yoga the Sadhaka
sets before himself the goal of conquering disease and decay, and,
with this aim in view, undertakes the arduous task of *kaya sadhana,* or the Culture of the Body, to make it invulnerable to
death by gaining control not only over respiration, circulation of
blood, digestion, and elimination with *pranayama* and *shatkarma,*
but also over the autonomic nervous system and the brain in
order to gain immortal life with a *siddha deha* or Perfect Body.
The idea of prolonging the life of the body for indefinite periods
was also prevalent among the Taoist sects of China, Tibetan
Tantrics, and alchemists of ancient times. There is no doubt that,
when benignly disposed in a healthy body, the awakening of
kundalini can lead to rejuvenation, prolongation of life, and
immunity to disease commensurate with the possibilities latent in
the human constitution. This might have happened in exceptional cases in the past. But lack of sufficient data about this
mighty mechanism, designed by nature for injecting a new life
into the human body, not only makes the enterprise directed to
activate it highly dangerous at this stage of our knowledge, but
also stands in the way of deriving all possible benefit from its
activity when it is aroused. Because of the extremely uncertain
nature of the experiment, it has been said about this Yoga that
the Sadhaka holds immortality in one hand and death in the
other. The lure of unfading youth, victory over death, miraculous
powers, and the capacity of enjoyment of the pleasures on earth
for cyclic periods of time has been, perhaps, one of the most

powerful factors in antiquity in attracting neophytes to the arduous enterprise of Hatha-Yoga. There are countless people even now, including men of learning, who have an inborn faith that such a possibility does exist in the occult systems of a religious discipline such as Yoga, not knowing, sometimes, that this faith springs from the promises that lie concealed in the natural Fountain of the Elixir of Life, *kundalini*.

Because of their stringent nature some of the practices of Hatha-Yoga have been kept secret and never divulged except to the initiates who, in the eyes of the preceptor, possessed the physical fitness and the presence of mind necessary to emerge from the ordeal safe and sound. Even with such rigorous training and strict body control only very few of the Sadhakas could stand the ordeal without succumbing to the severity of the trial. From this it is easy to gauge the magnitude of the risk involved for an ordinary individual in modern complex society, especially for one who has no practice in, nor even the possibility of gaining such complete control over the body as is envisaged in, the difficult *shatkarma* exercises. Even fearless anchorites, divested of all worldly responsibility and trained to perfection, often gave way before the rigor of the ordeal. The implication of this well-known aspect of Kundalini-Yoga, which is of paramount importance in understanding the biological basis of this cult, is often overlooked. The point that should have excited curiosity is that if there is a risk in the enterprise (and a whole system of body-control exercises has been devised to minimize that risk by manipulation of the visceral organs), it clearly indicates that the practice creates a disturbance in the body for which a certain state of preparedness and control over the vital organs is necessary. It is a matter of regret that because of the cloud of mistrust and suspicion under which this system has been laboring in the past, it has received less attention from the learned than it deserved. It is easy to understand that the risk mentioned and the disturbance guarded against, whether psychical or physical, could not be due to causes that have no material basis, because if such were the case the necessity for purely physical measures to combat the danger would not arise.

It is therefore obvious that the danger apprehended and the disturbances feared must be of a physical nature. The danger is particularly related to *pranayama*. In Hatha-Yoga practices, *pranayama* is the lever by which the serpent power is awakened. "Performed in the prescribed manner," says Hatha-Yoga Pradipika (2.41), "*pranayama* purifies the nerve-circuit enabling *prana* in good form to pierce (the mouth of) *susumna* and to enter through it." With the entry of *prana* in the central canal (*susumna*) the startling manifestations peculiar to Hatha-Yoga, but possible in other forms of Yoga also, begin to make their appearance in the body of the Sadhaka. The arduous types of *pranayama*, recommended in the books on Hatha-Yoga, are always attended by a certain amount of risk. There is not only a possibility of damage to the lung tissue, caused by overstrain, leading to disease, but danger to the safety of the nervous system as well. It is for this reason that special stress is laid in Hatha-Yoga manuals on beginning the exercises with restraint under the instructions of a competent Guru along with close adherence to a strict regimen in food and drink.

In his exposition Vacaspati Misra refers to *manu* (vi. 72), in which he says, "By restraints of breath one should burn up defects." In the Yoga-Sara-Sangraha (second part), it is said on the authority of Yoga-Vasistha that one who becomes proficient in performing *kumbhaka* (the retentive phase of *pranayama*) without resorting to the other two, that is the inhalation and the exhalation phases, can achieve anything he desires in the three worlds. The importance of *pranayama* as a means of achieving fixity of attention is admitted by Patanjali in i. 34 and ii. 53 of his Yoga-Sutras.

In the Hatha-Yoga system, however, combined with the *bandhas* and *mudras, pranayama* takes a more drastic and, at the same time, a more unnatural and precarious form. Its effect on the body of the Sadhaka, especially one not favored with a hardy and robust constitution, being often fraught with danger, particularly in the initial stages, the practice of *shatkarma* seems to have been introduced to give a tone to the system and to offset the injurious effects resulting from the overstrain and the disorganization caused in the body by the drastic exercise. "Proficiency in *shatkarma* before beginning the practice of *pranayama*," says Hatha-Yoga Pradipika, "is necessary for one who has excess of fat or phlegm in him. But for one who is free from these defects (has a harmonious state of the humors) *shatkarma* is not necessary." Since the standard of health demanded by a rigorous training of this kind is uncommon, recourse to *shatkarma* is almost always taken by those who devote themselves to Hatha-Yoga. The control over the visceral organs gained by it can always be used with advantage to combat disturbances in which the whole body, including the brain and the digestive system, is involved. Support for this view is again furnished by the unambiguous statements made in the Tantras that particular difficulty is experienced when *kundalini* pierces the three *granthis,* or knots, located at the *muladhara anahata,* and *ajna cakras,* especially the second one, commanding the heart and navel centers which, it is said, can cause great disorder and even disease.

If we now turn to the science of therapeutics for guidance in this matter we will find that the need to irrigate the large intestine or to empty the stomach arises in acute digestive disturbances, and the washing of the colon is sometimes resorted to in delirious conditions of the brain, caused by toxemia arising from a poisoned condition of the blood. This is exactly why these methods of purification of the internal organs were practiced by the ancient students of this Yoga, no doubt, after long experience and study of the symptoms caused by a sudden awakening of the serpent power. This means that, if the practices grouped under *shatkarma* are to be taken as an indication of the reactions caused in the body by *pranayama* or the arousal of *kundalini,* they provide strong evidence for the assumption that the exercises of Hatha-Yoga can lead to a sudden change in the organic

balance of the body of a type that can precipitate serious disturbances (of both a psychological and a physical nature), and it is
necessary to fight with extraordinary presence of mind and control over the digestive and other organs. With the enormous advances made in the knowledge of medicine and surgery, most of
the purposes served by these practices can now be achieved by
mechanical devices: stomach pump, enema, etc., but they fail in
one essential aspect, that is, the confidence and the will power
gained by the practitioner in the process of winning mastery over
his body by these methods.

It is known that the most critical period, when the constant
presence and guidance of the Guru is considered indispensable,
is the time of awakening. The Guru continues to supervise the
operation closely till the *ajna cakra* is reached. After this stage
the Sadhaka watches closely until the *ajna cakra* is reached. The
Sadhaka then enters the hierarchy of the accomplished ones, and
their relations as perceptor and disciple cease. Sometimes the
Guru even bows to the disciple at this point, in recognition of the
surpassing achievement. This ceremony of bowing to the disciple
at the end of the initiation ceremony of a neophyte, admitted to
the order, is even now performed by some ascetic sects in India
in imitation of the ancient custom. The Guru/disciple relationship ends at the sixth center, or the Cakra of Command, as
the Yogi is now guided by intuition and has access to a Fount
of Knowledge higher than that of any mortal Guru. The hazardous nature of the enterprise and the colossal nature of the task
that made the constant guidance of a preceptor necessary have
been often conveyed by the Yoga adepts of India in cryptic expressions like "diving deep in the ocean without getting wet" or
"making the frog dance before the serpent" or, as Lalla has said,
"submitting to thunder and lightening" or "being ground to
powder in a mill."

Pranayama is of several kinds. In the Yoga-Sutras of Patanjali
and in the Hatha-Yoga treatises three phases of the process are
recognized. First is *puraka,* that is, inhalation which is done by

closing either the right or the left nostril with the thumb and forefinger of one hand applied to the place. Then comes *kumbhaka,* or the retentive phase, when the inhaled air is retained inside for a certain duration of time. This is followed by *recaka,* or the exhalation of the breath through the other nostril. This makes one *pranayama.* The process is repeated either by inhaling again from the same nostril from which the breath has been expelled or from the one through which it was first inhaled. The duration of each phase is regulated either by repeating mentally the mystic syllable *Om* or any other Mantra, or by keeping count of time with the fingers of the other hand. The three phases are of the same or different durations. *Kumbhaka* may be done for a period twice or four times that of the *puraka,* and *recaka* twice or of the same duration as *puraka.* One form of *pranayama* is done by retaining the breath outside after it is expelled for a certain duration before another inhalation is done.

About the various methods of *pranayama,* as prescribed by different exponents, enough has been said to show that the ultimate objective is to reduce the rhythm of breathing to such an extent that it becomes hardly perceptible or, in the words of Vacaspati Misra, a bit of cotton held before the nostrils should remain unmoved in the flow of the breath. In the Yoga-Sara-Sangraha (second part) the place of precedence is allotted to *kumbhaka,* which can continue for months and years without *purama* and *recaka.* This is designated as *kevala kumbhaka,* and is known as the fourth *pranayama,* beyond count, time, and space. *Kevala kumbhaka* also finds mention in Yoga-ttatva Upanishad. With the attainment of proficiency in this *pranayama* the power to travel in space and other *siddhis,* it is said, come into the possession of the Sadhaka. Clearly, therefore, the aim of the practice is to diminish breathing to a degree that it appears that one is not breathing at all or, in other words, is apparently in a perennial *kumbhaka,* that is, in a state of suspended breathing. Whether the duration of *puraka, kumbhaka* and *recaka* are uniform or they are made to vary in a certain proportion, the effort of the Sadhaka is to be directed toward increasing the interval by slow degrees till an extremely reduced rhythm, working effortlessly, is attained.

The following observation of Mircea Eliade in his book, *Yoga, Immortality and Freedom*, dwelling on some of the effects caused by *pranayama*, is deserving of attention: "The Indian ascetics recognize four modalities of consciousness (in addition to the enstatic "state"): diurnal consciousness, consciousness in sleep with dreams, consciousness in sleep without dreams and 'Cataleptic consciousness.' By means of Pranayama, that is by increasingly prolonging inhalation and exhalation (the goal of the practice being to allow as long an interval as possible to pass between the two moments of respiration)—the Yogi can, then, penetrate all the modalities of consciousness. For the non-initiate there is discontinuity between these several modalities; thus he passes from the state of waking to the state of sleep unconsciously. The Yogi must preserve continuity of consciousness—that is he must penetrate each of these states with determination and lucidity."

By the term "cataleptic consciousness," Eliade refers to *turiya*, or the fourth state of consciousness, the other three being the states of wakefulness, dream, and dreamless sleep. According to the Indian scriptures, *turiya* is the state of self-knowledge or illumination in which the identity of the *Atman* and *Brahman* or *Jiva* or *Iswara* is realized. It is the indescribable state of existence experienced in the highest form of *samadhi* or the ecstatic "state," as Eliade calls it. The confusion seems to arise from the fact that he distinguishes between *samadhi* and *turiya* while, in actual fact, *turiya* is the modality of consciousness present in *asamprajnata, nirvikalpa,* or *nirbija samadhi,* and also characterizes the consciousness of a Jivan-Mukta, or one liberated in life. This is clear on the authority of Mandukya Upanishad (7) wherein it is said: "They consider the Fourth (that is *turiya*) to be that which is not conscious of the internal world nor conscious of the external world. . . . That is the Self and that is to be known." Again (in 12) it says: "The partless *Om* is the Fourth (*caturthah,* i.e., *turiya*)—beyond all conventional dealings, the limit of the negation of the phenomenal world, the auspicious and the non-dual. *Om* is thus the Self to be sure. He who knows thus enters the Self through the Self." The position has been clarified beyond doubt by Gaudapada in his Karika (i.14 and 15). "The earlier two (*visva* and *taijasa*) are endowed with dream and sleep, but *prajna* is endowed with dreamless sleep. People of firm conviction do not see either sleep or dream in *turiya.* . . . Dream belongs to one who sees falsely, and sleep to one who does not know Reality. When the two errors of these two are removed, one attains the state that is *turiya.*"

The point here is whether these four modalities of consciousness are characteristic of the embodied spirit or whether they have an independent existence of their own. The first three, it is hardly necessary to argue, have no independent existence, that is, they do not exist as cosmic planes of wakefulness, dreaming, and dreamless sleep, but represent different states of human consciousness. They are mutually exclusive, that is, as argued by Gaudapada, when one is dreaming he cannot be awake and when in dreamless slumber he can neither dream nor be awake. Similarly when one is awake he cannot dream, in the real sense of the term, nor can he be in dreamless slumber. It is, therefore, obvious that the moment a Yogi enters the dream state with lucidity, that is consciousness, dreaming must cease forthwith and when one enters the state of dreamless slumber it too must vanish instantly, for the simple reason that as darkness and light cannot exist together, in the same way the oblivion of the dream state and dreamless slumber cannot coexist with lucidity for any length of time. It might be contended that the so-called ecstatic "state" (*samadhi*), being a transhuman plane of consciousness, can "penetrate" the other three. In reply to this it is enough to point out that at the very moment when transhuman consciousness penetrates any modality of human consciousness it must at once transform and illumine it. It can neither assume the modality into which it enters nor coexist with it.

The point has been discussed at some length to show what grave misconceptions exist in respect of *samadhi* and the transcendent states of consciousness even among eminent scholars both in India and in other places. From this it is easy to infer the amount of error in the minds of the common people about these fascinating but still very little understood mental states. The terminology used by the ancient writers is sometimes so technical and difficult and the expositions are so varied that for those who have not had the experience it is extremely difficult to make even a remote mental picture of it. The conflicts and contradictions that occur as a result of this difficulty are, therefore, only natural. The experience of *samadhi* is not an artificial or extraneous mental condition, brought about by the suppression of thought, nor a magical state of perception that can "penetrate" into the dreamless and dream levels of the mind while retaining an awareness of the process, so that one continues to remain conscious that he is dreaming or in dreamless sleep all through the paradoxical episode. But it denotes a transformation of the whole personality—dream state, dreamless slumber, waking and all—a marvelous rise to higher planes of consciousness, the emergence of an effulgent, sublime inner being (called *divya deha*, or divine body, by the ancients) which persists through all the three states of waking, dreaming, and dreamless sleep in the same way as the normal personality of an individual persists through them.

Pratyahara is defined by Patanjali (II. 54) as the withdrawal of senses from their objects in conformity with the restrictions imposed by the mind. In his commentary on this Sutra, Vyasa explains *pratyahara* in this way: "When there is no conjunction with their own objects, the organs in imitation of the mind-stuff, as it is in itself, become, as it were, restricted. When the mind-stuff is restricted, like the mind-stuff they become restricted; and do not, like the subjugation of the senses, require any further aid. Just as when the Queen-bee flies up, the bees fly up after her, and when she settles down, they settle down after her. So when the mind-stuff is restricted, the organs are restricted. Thus

there is the withdrawal of the senses." Yoga-Sara-Sangraha, citing
the authority of Narada Purana, defines *pratyahara* as the withdrawal of senses from all the objects in which they are engrossed.
"The Yoga practitioner," it says, "who applies himself to meditation (*dhyana*) without first subduing his senses can only be considered as unintelligent, as the meditation of such a person can
never bear fruit." Gheranda Samhita (iv. 3. 4. 5) defines *pratyahara* as the withdrawal of mind from honor and opprobrium,
from what is good to hear and what is not good to hear, from
what is odorous and malodorous, from sweet, sour and bitter,
from any form of sound, smell or taste by which the mind is
drawn to bring it back under the control of the Self (*Atman*).
The Bhagavad-Gita (ii. 57. 58) describes the state of one observing *pratyahara* in these words: "Stable is the mind of him who,
unattached to everything, meets good and evil without rejoicing
at the one and feeling revulsion at the other. . . . When a man
like a tortoise, which draws in its limbs from all directions, withdraws his senses from the objects of desire then he attains to a
stable state of mind."

"The first five limbs of Yoga, from *yama* to *pratyahara*," says
Yoga-Sara-Sangraha, "are for the control of the body, *prana* and
the senses and the other three limbs, *dharana, dhyana* and *samadhi* for the control of *citta* (consciousness)." Divested of the
mystical and magical coloring with which some writers on Yoga
try to invest these practices, *dharana* is simple concentration on
certain susceptible regions of the body or on some object, with
a mental content relating to some aspect of Divinity, to the
supernatural or the numinous. *Dhyana* is deeper concentration
persisting for a longer time and *samadhi* is the absorption of
the mercurial mind in the contemplation of the Self. According
to Patanjali (1.2.3.4) "When the mind-stuff is restricted then
the Seer (that is, the Self) abides in himself. At other times It
(the Self) takes the same form as the fluctuations (of the mind-
stuff)." A man deeply engrossed in study or in painting or in any
other absorbing occupation is in a state of concentration. A classi-

cal example of absorbed concentration, cited in Yoga-Sara-San-graha, refers to the mental condition of an arrow-maker who is so engrossed in his work that he fails to see the king passing by.

"Binding the mind-stuff to a place is fixed attention (*dharana*)" says Patanjali in the Yoga-Sutras (3.1). Commenting on it, Vyasa says: "Binding of the mind-stuff, only in so far as it is a fluctuation, to the navel or to the heart lotus or to the light within the head or to the tip of the nose or to the tip of the tongue or to other places of the same kind or to an external object—this is fixed attention." *Dharana, dhyana* and *samadhi* are, in actual fact, the three successive phases of one single effort directed toward making the attention one-pointed. When *dharana* becomes continuous it is *dhyana.* Vacaspati Misra in his exposition of Sutra 3.2 of the Yoga-Sutras, cites a passage from Vishnu Purana in which *dhyana* is explained in these words: "An uninterrupted succession of presented ideas single-in-intent upon His (the Deity's) form without desire for anything else, that, O King, is contemplation (*dhyana*)." In other words *dhyana* is the continuous flow of thought on one single object to the exclusion of all other thoughts. According to the Sarva-Sarsana-Sangrha, "the continual flow of thought in one place, resting on the object to be contemplated, and avoiding all incongruous thought" is *dhyana.* The same view is expressed in Isvar-Gita quoted in Yoga-Sara-Sangraha.

Studied from a rational angle, the practice of *dharana* and *dhyana,* as expounded in the Yoga-Sutras and other ancient books has nothing "mysterious" or "magical" or "mystical" about them. *Dhyana,* deep meditation, connotes fixity of attention on one object and this connotation has come unaltered from the Vedic period in India. It is, of course, the intensity with which concentration of mind is practiced and the will and perseverance behind the practice which are decisive in achieving success in the enterprise. The various exercises of Yoga including *asana, pranayama,* and *pratyahara* lend a potency to concentration which is not possible in other ways. It is the power of *ekagarta,* or one-pointedness of thought, which is effective in stimulating the center of para-normal consciousness in the brain, commanding *susumna,* where on the awakening of the *kundalini,* the Flame of Super-consciousness burns with transporting effect. The important point to be kept in mind is that *dharana* and *dhyana* are not ends in themselves, but means to an end and that end is the excitation of the Transcendent center in the head. It is with the aim of stimulating this region and *susumna* that fixity of attention on one of the susceptible nerve-junctions, as for instance, the navel, or the heart, or the place between the eyebrows, or the palate, or the crown of the head is recommended by the ancient writers on Yoga. In his commentary on Yoga-Sutra 3. 1, Vyasa recommends concentration on the navel, heart, or light in the head for the same reason.

Dharana, dhyana and *samadhi* are the three last steps toward the attainment of a fuller and richer life. In *samadhi* the mental flux becomes entirely restricted and the stream of thought becomes one with the object contemplated. In every spiritual practice the object kept before the mind being either the Deity with or without form or the Self or the Guru or some transporting object, like the lotus, or any iconographic representation, pre-scribed for meditation, complete absorption of mind in the object plainly signifies a transformation in the interior of the Sadhaka. In other words, it denotes the development of a new quality in his own consciousness which, assuming the image of the Deity or the Self or a lotus or a light, keeps the attention of the Sadhaka from wandering this way or that, and holds it completely engrossed in contemplation in the same way that a magnet holds a piece of iron tightly attached to it by the sheer force of attraction. It is the development of this alluring quality in his consciousness that keeps the Yogi entranced for hours without any sign of fatigue and with a beatific expression on his face. The arrest of thought in *samadhi* does not occur because of the restraint exercised by the Yogi, but, primarily, because the mind is rapt in the contemplation of a fascinating inner state which may intervene either by imperceptible degrees or suddenly during the practice of *dhyana*. This is Yoga, the state of rapturous union between the fluctuating mind-stuff and the ravishing Universe of Consciousness which now begins to loom large on the mental horizon of the Sadhaka.

This is the reason why repeated mention is made in all Indian scriptures and books on Yoga of the incomparable bliss of *samadhi*. The ceaselessly repeated expression *Sat-Cit-Ananda*, the keyword of Vedanta to signify the Ineffable, meaning Existence-Consciousness-Bliss, is symbolic of the enrapturing trans-human state of consciousness experienced in *samadhi*. "He, the Self-existent Being is verily of the nature of Bliss," says the Taittiriyopanishad (ii.7). "Having attained this Bliss one becomes blessed." That the aim of *samadhi* is Cosmic Consciousness is expressed by Atmopanishad (3) in these words: "Now about the Parmatman: Verily He is to be worshipped according to the precepts of the Vedas. And He (reveals himself) to one who, through the Yoga of Pranayama, Pratyahara and Samadhi or through reasoning meditates on the Adhyatma. He is like the banyan seed or like the Syamaka grain: conceived of as being as subtle as a hundred-thousandth fraction of the point of a hair, and so forth. He cannot be grasped or perceived. He is not born. He does not die. He is neither dried up nor burnt, nor shaken, nor pierced, nor severed. He is beyond all qualities, the Witness, eternal, pure, of the essence of the indivisible, one only, subtle, without components, without taint, without egoism, devoid of sound, touch, taste, sight and smell, devoid of doubt, without expectation. He is all-pervading, unthinkable, indescribable. He purifies the unclean and the defiled. He is without action. He has no Samaskaras. He is the Purusa who is called the Parmatman."

Bliss (*ananda*) with an indescribable state of Being is the keynote of the *samadhi* attained in Raja-Yoga, Laya-Yoga, Mantra-Yoga, Hatha-Yoga, Jnana-Yoga, Bakhti-Yoga, Karma-Yoga, and also the attribute of the Supreme, conceived by Vedantists, Saivites, Sakts, Tantric Buddhists, Sahajas, Vaisnavites, and the rest. It is obvious from this that *pranayama, dhyana, niskama karma* (desireless action), *jnana, bhakti,* and *kundalini* ultimately lead to the same mental condition. Are not the ecstasy resulting from concentrated bliss, said to be far more intense than the highest transport experienced in the climax of the embrace of love, and the inexpressibly marvelous nature of the Vision sufficient baits to keep the attention of the Yogi riveted for the time being, completely immobilized and transfixed by the sheer transport of the experience? Just as a man, intensely watching an entrancing drama, becomes at times oblivious of his surroundings and does not even hear when spoken to and, by identifying himself completely with the play, ceases to pay attention to his body and the impressions coming from his senses, in the same way, multiplied a dozenfold, a Yogi, rapt in *samadhi,* becomes oblivious to his body, his senses, and the world to such an extent that even loud noises and other distracting factors fail to interrupt the state of utter absorption in which, for the time being, he is immersed. The difference beween *dhyana* and *samadhi,* according to the Yoga-Sara-Sangraha, lies in this: violent sensory impression coming from outside can cause interruption in the state of absorption attained in the former, but fail to do so in the latter. It is about this state of ecstatic contemplation, when the mind is completely identified with the object contemplated, that the Knower, Known, and the process of Knowing, it is said, become one. In this condition with but a vestige of the ego left, even if he wishes it, the entranced Yogi cannot withdraw his mind from the state of rapt contemplation till the ecstasy is over. The only method of recalling Paramhamsa Rama-Krishna from his ecstatic trances, it is said, was to pronounce a name of the Lord or some Mantra into his ear.

The difficulty experienced by intellect in understanding the real nature of *samadhi* is reflected in this passage from Mircea Eliade's *Yoga, Immortality and Freedom** ". . . It would be

*Pantheon, New York, 1958.

wrong to regard this mode of being of the Spirit as a simple 'trance' in which consciousness was emptied of all content. Non-differentiated ecstasies are not 'absolute emptiness.' The 'state' and the 'knowledge' simultaneously expressed by this term refer to a total absence of objects in consciousness, not to a consciousness absolutely empty. For, on the contrary, at such a moment consciousness is saturated with a direct and total intuition of being. As Madhava says, 'Nirodha (final arrest of all psychomental experience) must not be imagined as nonexistence, but rather as the support of a particular condition of the spirit.' It is the enstasis of total emptiness, without sensory content or intellectual structure, an unconditioned state that is no longer 'experience' (for there is no further relation between consciousness and the world), but 'revelation.' Intellect (buddhi), having accomplished its mission, withdraws, detaching itself from the purusa and returning into prakrti. The Self remains free, autonomous; it contemplates itself. 'Human' consciousness is suppressed; that is, it no longer functions, its constituent elements being reabsorbed into the primordial substance. The Yogin attains deliverance; like a dead man, he has no more relation with life; he is 'dead in life.' He is the 'Jivan-Mukta,' the 'liberated in life.' He no longer lives in time and under the domination of time, but in an eternal present, in the *nunc stans* by which Boethius defined eternity. . . ."

The difficulty and the misconceptions arise from the fact that the state of "trance" or oblivion to the world is considered to be an unalterable characteristic of *samadhi*. This, in its turn, naturally creates the idea that during this condition human consciousness and human thoughts are completely suppressed and the Self or, in other words, the Light behind the intellect and mind, now free from all distractions, contemplates itself. It has been explained that if ego-consciousness were entirely suppressed the Yogi cannot bring the least recollection of what is experienced in *samadhi* when he returns to his normal condition. Second, what is more explicit, a perennial *samadhi,* as in the case of a Jivan-Mukta, can never be possible. If the elimination of the human condition and the suppression of the intellect and mind are an invariable feature of *samadhi,* how can a Jivan-Mukta, at all attend to the needs of the body and survive for any length of time? The remark of Eliade that "the Yogin attains deliverance; like a dead man he has no more relations with life: he is 'dead in life' " is far from the reality. The highest products of Yoga in India, Abhinava Gupta, Sankara, Ramanuja, Kabir, Nanak, and others, were all men of action, with exceptional mental gifts and intellectual acumen, who brought glory to the land by their peerless contribution to the spiritual thought of mankind. For a correct understanding of Yoga, therefore, a new orientation is necessary, especially in the West. *Samadhi* can occur both with entrancement and oblivion to the world and also in full wakefulness as a normal feature of a higher state of consciousness. How this apparently paradoxical situation comes about will be explained in another work. But even in the case of the former, as for example in the instance of Ramakrishna, Chaitanya, and others, as also in some of the Christian mystics one is never "dead to the world" but actively engaged, more actively, perhaps, than is the case with normal men, in the moral and spiritual enlightenment of mankind.

6

Kundalini, the Key to Cosmic Consciousness

Before attempting to offer an explanation for the indescribable mystical state let us see how far the usually accepted idea of Grace can cover the varied manifestations of the phenomenon. In the utterances of prophets, mystics and saints themselves the factor of Grace in the achievement is again and again emphasized. The belief is of great antiquity, almost as old as religious experience itself, and is repeatedly expressed in the religious literature of the world. Among the Buddhists the ever-abiding Buddha is substituted for God. Considering the fact that from the very beginning the human mind has attributed the existence of all phenomena, inexplicable to it, to the agency of supernatural entities or divine beings, it is no wonder that for the still more incomprehensible mystical experience an added degree of divine favor has been thought to be a sufficient explanation for it. Until very recent times intractable diseases were often ascribed to the maleficent influence of evil stars or spirits, gods or goddesses even by the civilized populations of Europe and Asia, and exorcism or propitiation was resorted to, sometimes with adverse effects, to cure the malady. In India, even after the discovery of vaccination and with the full knowledge that it provides an effective safeguard against the disease, many credulous people side by side with the inoculation, present the customary offering to the goddess Shitalla, the presiding deity of smallpox, to appease her. Similar practices are common in other lands also, and the practice of wearing amulets against bad luck and disease still continues in Europe among a large number of people.

In the light of this tendency of the human mind, ascribing the vicissitudes of life to the favor or disfavor of God or other divine beings, which was much more pronounced in the comparatively darker ages of the past, the factor of divine Grace to account for the mystical state was the only possible and reasonable explanation to offer for the extraordinary condition. Thus in the Svetasvatara Upanishad it is said that Svetasvatara came to realize *Brahman* through austerities and the grace of God. Katha-Upanishad goes a step further when it declares that neither by studying nor by listening to the scriptures can the Self be realized and that realization can be gained only when the Self desires to manifest itself. In the Gita the importance of grace is constantly stressed and in the last chapter Krishna promises liberation to Arjuna if he eschews all striving and comes to Him alone for refuge. Connected with the doctrine of Grace is also the stress laid on the imperative need of a really qualified preceptor or Guru among all the mystical sects of India, Tantric Buddhists, and Sufis. The homage to be paid to the teacher who initiates one into the knowledge of *Brahman* is emphasized to a high degree in the Tantras. The Guru is compared to God and even substituted for Him, and it is held that only through the flash of intuition, passing from the Guru to the disciple, like the passing of a flame from one lighted candle to another, can the transcendent state be attained.

Among the religious-minded, even during these days of unprecedented material progress, when satisfactory explanations for many of the hitherto obscure phenomena of nature have been furnished by science, an attitude of solicitation and surrender toward the Almighty Source of all creation at times of extreme mental stress, grave danger and in serious illness, where the success of human efforts remains in doubt, is common among both the scholars and the laity. This healthy instinctive gesture of

the human mind, still enveloped in the mystery of its own existence and always at the mercy of gigantic natural forces, acts as
an inherent safety device to keep a frustrated sensitive mind from
giving way completely under the strain. To ascribe the mysterious process of illumination of a seeker when he comes face to
face with the awe-inspiring, indescribable phenomenon within
himself, to the Grace of God or the divine in himself or to the
favor of the Guru, has, therefore, been a natural confirmation
to this instinctive tendency of the human mind. The object of
the quest being God or the *Brahman* or the Self or some Deity
the conclusion was natural that the encounter could not take
place without His or Its concurrence and favor.

Grace has, therefore, come to hold a very important place
among the seekers after transcendent experience of all shades of
thought, of all religions and creeds, and of all epochs. Until the
whole phenomenon of religious experience is explained to the
satisfaction of the intellect, the idea of Grace will and must continue to hold sway in the present or in a modified form over the
minds of the people. It should, however, be obvious to every keen
observer that the various factors involved in every kind of genuine mystical experience are so strongly marked and persistent
that, apart from the factor of grace, conformity to some still
obscure biological and psychic laws is indicated as a precondition
to the supreme experience. For instance, we find that purity of
conduct, a high degree of morals, love of God or other Deity,
constant thought of the end in view, and a passionate longing for
the experience are necessary for success in the undertaking. So
are self-denial, control of passions, and a heart aflame with the
love of fellow beings. Grace is in a way a responsive gesture from
the Unseen, a sign of assent from Divinity or a sort of permit
from the Almighty Cosmic Forces to a deserving aspirant to
approach the Ineffable, normally beyond the reach of ordinary
mortals. But the very fact that certain norms of conduct have
been prescribed for the guidance of seekers by every religion and
every esoteric creed is a clear indication that Grace itself is de-

pendent on a number of factors that must attend the efforts of
the seeker.

Conformity to a certain spiritual discipline betokens the need
for preparation and effort, a tuning of the mind and body to the
demands of a higher plane of life. At the present state of our
knowledge what makes Grace an essential ingredient of transcendent experience is the incontrovertible fact that in the first
place the supreme vision is granted only to an infinitely small
minority out of the countless millions who strive for it, some
even with a greater regard for the higher standards of conduct
on the path than those who unexpectedly attain the crown, and,
second, because the highest experience from the remotest past
has come naturally to a few as a heaven-bestowed gift from their
very birth. This aspect of the problem presents an almost irrefutable argument in favor of the position that Grace is indispensable for salvation, except when we recollect that in the case of
genius, superior mental gifts and psychic powers as well as the
possession of the talent are determined by birth, and the efforts of
but a few in a vast number of competitors fructify much more
rapidly or bear a more abundant and richer harvest than the
others.

If we accept Grace as the sole factor responsible for success
in any spiritual enterprise, we have then to concur with the view
of those who consider success in worldly undertakings as a mark
of divine favor or reward for previous *karmas*. Birth into an
affluent and well-placed family, providing far greater opportuni-
ties for a life of happiness and prosperity, or a superior physical
endowment at birth, enabling one to shine in athletics and sports
and to outshine other equally hard-working contestants, should
also then be ascribed to the same cause. Marginal escapes in acci-
dents, cure of patients declared to be past human help, unexpected strokes of luck, winning in gambles and lotteries and
other similar occurrences which, in absence of a rational explanation, we are accustomed to ascribe to chance should also then fall
into the same category. When this is conceded then every occur-

rence which we cannot explain will have to be considered as God-ordained. In fact this is the usual attitude of mind of the devoutly religious. That not a leaf can move without command is an idea common to almost all great religions of the world.

Considered from this aspect, we can say with justice that all that happens in this universe, from the movement of atoms to the motions of colossal suns and gigantic sidereal systems, proceeds from the invisible Power that has brought this mighty creation into existence. As man is but a helpless spectator of a mighty drama, covering the whole of space, in which humanity occupies no higher position than that of a colony of microbes, or a small pebble on the bed of a vast ocean filled with rocks and boulders from end to end, always impotent before the mighty cosmic forces that sweep round him, regardless of his choice, he has only two ways open to explain the situation, either the whole drama is a monstrous play of lifeless forces ruled by laws in which his existence is a matter of accident, or the stupendous performance proceeds from an Almighty Intelligence, which ordains and rules all its activity. From this point of view everything that happens in the cosmos, every action we perform, every breath we draw, every pain we suffer, every joy we taste, every failure and success we face all come from God.

For such an attitude, there should be no difference in the success achieved in a worldly project or in a victory gained in the spiritual realm. Both are equally due to divine favor. But for one who desires to probe into the nature of things, to satisfy the cravings of the intellect, the phenomenon of illumination is as much a matter for investigation as any other phenomenon of nature. In spite of the fact that the robust constitution of a powerful athlete is determined to a large extent by his birth, no one can deny the fact that regular exercise, coupled with a healthy mode of life, develops his arms, thighs, chest and legs in a way that gives a distinctive shape to his body, a symmetry to his limbs, and an agility to his movements not found in those who have not undergone the training. He becomes capable of prodi-

gious feats of strength not possible for ordinary men. We do not
yet understand the whole process as to how the nerves and muscles
coordinate to fashion the muscular body of a strong man, but we
are in no doubt about the fact that proper exercise, nourishing
diet, and a healthy way of life are necessary to bring this about.

In the same way we know that apart from those who are spiritually gifted from their birth (as for instance in the case of the
South Indian saint, Jnaneshwar, who wrote a commentary on
the Gita at the age of sixteen, ministered to the spiritual needs of
countless people, and left an inspiring collection of poems before
passing away at the age of twenty-one), some sort of mental discipline, some kind of spiritual exercise, attention to morals, austerity with a passionate desire for the experience, nobility of
action and elevated conduct have always formed a part of the
efforts of those who achieved success in their spiritual quest.
Even in the case of the born mystic and seer, as if a natural
accompaniment to the condition, almost all these characteristics,
it has been found, are usually present from a very early age in
the majority of such people. In the light of these facts it would
be as incorrect to say that success in spiritual endeavor is purely
an act of Grace as it would be to ascribe the triumph of an
athlete merely to his birth, without taking into account the other
factors which contributed to the development necessary for
success.

A study of the lives of medieval saints and mystics, in both the
East and the West, makes it abundantly clear that a certain
norm of conduct and behavior, certain distinctive mental traits
and certain peculiar modes of thought and action have characterized all of them, without a single exception; but unfortunately
due to the fact that the biological factors underlying this condition have not been understood thus far, no attention has been
paid to the classification and study of this outstanding class of
men. Had this been done it would not have been difficult to
locate the factors responsible for the mental condition exhibited
by them, and to a lesser degree possessed by millions and millions

of people with inherent mystical tendencies, living in different parts of the earth today, irrespective of their religious belief and faith. It would have been found that, although there is no gainsaying the fact that some still unintelligible factors play a decisive role in the attainment of the final state of enlightenment, such as the as yet little understood factors determining the birth of human beings, there is a basic similarity not only in their temperament and behavior but also in the ultimate condition, the vision, and the ecstasy. This clearly indicates the existence of a new form of psychic activity in their systems, about which they are in the dark, like the play of erotic passions at the age of puberty in those brought up strictly in a cloistered environment which is, sometimes, the cause of mystification to them.

It is, therefore, obvious that though indispensable until the law underlying the phenomenon is thoroughly understood, the doctrine of Grace does not explain all aspects of the problem. If Grace is the sole arbitrator in man's search for the Divine how does it happen that some possess the gift from birth while others gain it only after years of rigid self-discipline and sacrifice? If we attribute this difference to the effect of *karma* it means eliminating Grace, since in that case *karma* becomes the decisive factor, and if we attribute it to the will of God we then impute arbitrariness and partiality to Him. The explanation offered by some scholars that mystical experience is a plunge into the subconscious is as correct as it would be to say that the ecstatic condition is only a realistic state of daydreaming. It is well known that clever tapping of the subconscious, attempted by present-day psychologists, does not often reveal an edifying or elevating spectacle. There is too much of the crude, the grotesque, and the animal in it. The lower passions and urges are found parading there in a state of utter nudity. Even in the case of those who, in the subconscious depths reached in a state of hypnosis, furnish incontestable proof of clairvoyance, memory of former births, or precognition, there is no elevation of personality, no blissful encounter with the Well-spring of Life, no taste of deathlessness and no intuitive flashes of eternal truths. It is a probe into the recesses of mind, no doubt, but of a mind which is the cause of our bondage and pain, the thin vapory envelope of our thoughts, passions, and fancies, the illusive veil of *maya* that hides the stupendous, undifferentiated ocean of egoless and deathless Consciousness, which the seers of the Upanishads called the *Brahman* or simply *That*. It is a historical fact that almost all the top-rank Yoga adepts in India have been men of outstanding intellectual attainments and they are all known by the harvest of their genius, the monumental works they have left behind. Such a bloom of the higher faculties of mind could never have been possible by an unnatural way of life combined with practices which aimed only at the annihilation of thought.

Patanjali himself says that when the suppression of the modifications of the mind-stuff is accomplished, "Then the seer (that is the Self) abides in himself" (i.3). As for the means to be adopted for the restriction of these fluctuations, he says (i.12): "This restriction is by (means of) practice and passionlessness." Commenting on it, Vyasa writes: "The so-called river of the mind-stuff whose flow is in both directions, flows toward good and flows toward evil. Now when it is borne onward to isolation (*kaivalya*), downward toward discrimination, then it is flowing unto good, when it is borne onward to the whirlpool of existence, downward toward nondiscrimination then it is flowing unto evil. In these cases the stream toward objects is damned by passionlessness and the stream toward discrimination has its flood-gates opened by practice in discriminatory knowledge." For a proper understanding of the Yoga expounded by Patanjali, and for that matter of any system of Yoga or religious discipline that makes use of concentration as a stepping-stone to higher spheres of consciousness, it is of paramount importance to bear in mind that the object is not to create a blank or a void by a complete stoppage of the process of thinking, but to change its direction from the outer gross world to the inner subtle one. This change of direction does not imply immersion into reveries and daydreaming, but the complete absorption of thought into and its identification with the well-spring of Consciousness, the Self, which, shining by Its own light, becomes increasingly conscious of Itself through practice, until It completely overshadows the world perceived by the senses. The mind then freed from the domination of desires and sensory impression remains rapt in the contemplation of the marvelous, extremely fascinating inner world.

How in the light of these facts can it be admitted that *samadhi* itself results in the cessation of thought, caused by intense concentration or by a diminished flow of blood to the brain, or by the stoppage or slowing down of the breath? Had the phenomenon been confined to the practice of *dhyana* or Hatha-Yoga only, even then the solution would provide insurmountable difficulties in the way of its acceptance by a rational mind. But when we find that the exercise of intellectual discrimination, selfless action, constant thought of Divinity, passionate devotion and, above all, merely a gesture from the Unseen in the form of Grace can bring about the mystic state, the whole problem assumes a different aspect altogether. It becomes obvious that all the current explanations offered for this condition do not, in these circumstances, provide a satisfactory answer to the riddle. There must be some other factor underlying and common to all these which exercises a decisive function in the attainment of the divine objective.

It is a commonly observed fact that the normal human consciousness is able to apply itself only to a limited field of observation at one time, and this law operates in sleep and hypnotic conditions also. For instance, while reading a paper we can scan only one word and one line at a given instant and not have all the words and all the lines of that page before our mind at the same time. Similarly while trying to imagine the colossal body of the sun, our largest picture of it can only correspond to the widest landscape seen, and can never exceed the limits of the mental horizon present in us; although the sun is millions of times the size of earth, all we see at one time from horizon to

horizon is but an infinitesimal part of the earth. The experience
of *samadhi,* as described by Yogis and saints, is a plunge into the
Infinite, a dive into the plumbless depths of an unbounded Conscious Ocean or the vision of an all-pervading Omnipotent Being,
or the face-to-face encounter with a personified God, of unlimited
power, in a halo of infinite glory, unlike anything seen on earth.

In all the genuine phenomena of this kind, the effect on the
visionary has been always stunning, and the experience has been
repeated, with variations of course, but always with a powerful
impact on the mind. The question is: How can this occasional
virtual metamorphosis of consciousness be explained in terms
of the solutions suggested? Either the whole subject is delusive and
the vision is only an overpowering hallucination, in which case
the inquiry need not proceed any further, or the phenomenon
is the outcome of an alteration in consciousness, resulting from
an alteration in the functioning of the brain. Arrest of thought
can at the most tend to keep the consciousness unruffled or, in
other words, it can cut off the impressions coming from the senses
and keep the flame of awareness absolutely steady for some time,
but it cannot enlarge the capacity of consciousness to such a
degree as to cause a staggering effect on the individual, wafted
to a new plane of being, to infinity and immortality. Unless there
occurs a radical transformation in the power of cognition of the
observer himself, allowing him to compare his former state with
the vision seen, the mystic state, as described by great Yogis and
mystics, is not possible. The consciousness will continue to have,
even in the condition of stillness of thought, the same limited
capacity as is allowed to it by the brain.

The argument that in the condition of *samadhi* consciousness
is dissociated from the brain and can, therefore, be realized in
all its majesty and universal character is not valid for the simple
reason that not infrequently both in the mystical state, occurring
spontaneously, and in *samadhi,* brought about by Yoga, the Deity
is apprehended as a personified Being, as in the case of *Vaishnava*
saints, Sufis, and Western mystics, which is not possible without

the agency of the brain. Even in the case of *nirvi-kalpa samadhi,* which is considered to be the highest state of illumination, the Yogi brings back the memory of the transmundane experience, when he comes again to his normal state, an impossible achievement unless the memory is awake all the time, demonstrating conclusively the continuing activity of the brain. There is no escape from the position that the rapturous descriptions of the ecstatic vision, described by those who had the supreme experience, could be possible only when they could retain a recollection of it in the normal state, establishing thereby a link between what they underwent in the trance condition and in their normal consciousness. This shows that in some way the surface consciousness continues to function in both conditions. If this were not the case the experience would leave no impression on the mind of the Yogi, as happens in syncope or deep sleep of which one has no recollection on awakening.

The view that the ego-consciousness completely ceases to operate at the time of mystical flight is contradicted by the accounts of the experience left by mystics, Yoga saints, and others, which clearly indicates that, even in such cases where the body shows all the outer signs of insensibility, the ecstatic state is still sufficiently alert to recall a memory of the extraordinary occurrence on returning to the normal state. "The Soul," says St. Teresa of Avila,* "neither sees, hears, nor understands anything while this state lasts; but this is usually a very short time, and seems to the soul even shorter than it really is. God visits the soul in a way that prevents it doubting when it comes to itself that it has been in God and God in it; and so firmly is it convinced of this truth that, though years may pass before this state recurs, the soul can never forget it nor doubt its reality. . . . But you will say, how can the soul see and comprehend that she is in God and God in her, if during this union she is not able either to see or understand? I reply, that she does not see it at the time, but that afterwards she perceives it clearly: not by a vision, but by a certitude

* *The Way of Perfection,* Newman Book Shop, Westminster, Maryland, 1948.

which remains in the heart which God alone can give." Here is an account of one of his *samadhis* given by Rama-Krishna Paramahamsa himself: "One day I found that my mind was soaring high in *samadhi* along a luminous path. It soon transcended the stellar universe and entered the subtler region of ideas. As it ascended higher and higher, I found on both sides of the way ideal forms of gods and goddesses. The mind then reached the outer limits of that region, where a luminous barrier separated the sphere of relative existence from that of the Absolute. Crossing that barrier, the mind entered the transcendent realm, where no corporeal being was visible. Even the gods dared not look into that sublime realm, and were content to keep their seats far below. But the next moment I saw seven venerable sages seated there in *samadhi*. It occurred to me that these sages must have surpassed not only men but even the gods in knowledge and holiness, in renunciation and love. Lost in admiration, I was reflecting on their greatness, when I saw a portion of that undifferentiated luminous region condense into the form of a divine child. . . ."

There is no denying the fact that in the case of *samadhi* brought about by Hatha-Yoga a deathlike state of the body can ensue as a result of more or less complete cessation of vital functions, caused by the almost complete interruption of breathing. The deathlike trance sometimes occurs naturally, as in the case of born mystics. But even in these cases the memory is partially active, since if this were not so, the Hatha-Yoga could not retain the memory of their visions. It is, therefore, obvious that the brain actively participates in inducing transcendent conditions of consciousness in a way which is a mystery at present. In some kinds of Hatha-Yoga *samadhi,* the Yogi loses all consciousness and, on returning to the normal state, has no recollection whatsoever of what he underwent in the trance. Yogis of this category demonstrate their mastery over their bodies by allowing themselves to be buried underground for days and even weeks. The astounding nature of this feat has led some present-day scholars to link superconsciousness with a cataleptic condition of the body, and they expect one with a transhuman state of consciousness to be able to stop his breathing and suspend his heart action, making the body inert and cold, that is, corpselike in appearance. This is an entirely erroneous position which we shall discuss at length elsewhere. Here it is enough to say that a corpselike condition supervenes only in some cases of Hatha-Yogis and not in Yogis in general, and among the former only a few attain to the supreme state of Transcendent Consciousness.

The fallacy of the notion that the arrest of thought can magically open the door to the Divine has already been pointed out. No method employed by man to experience a vision of the Transcendent Reality can ever be successful unless the human consciousness itself is developed to an extent where it can apprehend supersensory realms. Millions of Sadhus in India practice meditation for as much as twelve hours a day, and sit in the yogic posture even during the night, supporting their head and arms, while maintaining their erect position, on a flat piece of wood held aloft by a rod fastened to its middle, its other end planted firmly on the ground. They continue the practice for years without ever attaining *samadhi*. There is some mysterious element that has eluded the grasp not only of the adepts of the past but also the scholars of today, which must be present in all cases of a successful termination of the Yoga practice. The ancient masters, fully cognizant of the fact that in this enterprise success crowns the efforts of hardly one out of thousands of aspirants, attribute the anomaly to the effect of past *karma*, an explanation which they offer for the other inequalities of life also. But even admitting the operation of the law of *karma*, we have to accept the possibility that there must be some lack in the psychosomatic organization of the bodies of those who fail in this undertaking even after the most strenuous lifelong efforts to achieve a higher state of consciousness. Even those who believe implicitly in the law of *karma* do not hesitate to ascribe to a mediocre or inferior condition of the brain or to some defect in the body the failure of those who never shine intellectually or never acquire a strong physique, in spite of constant efforts made to achieve distinction in either. When on the physical plane, with belief in *karma,* in order to account for the absence of success in the efforts of the inferior condition of the brain, or the flaw in the construction of the body, is fully recognized, why should not failure in a spiritual effort also be ascribed to its temporal cause, that is to some lack in the mental and physical constitution of the Sadhaka about which we are in the dark at present?

In ancient Indian scriptures one of the factors responsible for success in spiritual endeavors is held to be the predominance of the *sattva* element, tending to a harmonized condition of the body and the mind which clearly points to the dependence of the experience on a certain favorable condition of the organism. Even among the sattvic aspirants success falls to the share of one out of hundreds. The ancient masters selected their disciples with the utmost care, always according preference to the purest and the most earnest among those who sought guidance from them. But in spite of this hardly one out of them all achieved the state of illumination and made not only himself but his Guru also immortal by his outstanding brilliance. The predominance of the *sattva* element, mentioned in the Gita, does not explain the reason for failures among the Sattvics in whom the percentage of success is very low. What then are the factors indispensable for genuine mystical experience? Since none of the solutions offered for transcendent conditions of consciousness is able to bear close scrutiny, and at the same time it is impossible to deny the phenomenon in consideration of the overwhelming evidence, it becomes necessary to place religion and transcendent religious experience on a solid foundation, beyond the shadow of uncertainty and doubt that hangs over it today, and to locate the mysterious factor which is responsible for all their enormously varied manifestations from prehistoric times to the present day.

Those who fear that a thorough analysis of religion and transcendent truths is not desirable, since scriptural knowledge is beyond the probe of reason and must always remain above it to avoid profanation, are inviting the very catastrophe which they dread. If faith is a mere bubble, liable to burst with only a pin-prick, it would be far better to make the prick sooner and watch the reaction, rather than that it should continue to exist as a hollow mass of vapory thought liable to burst and spread ruin around it at any time. The custodians of various faiths of mankind are often loath to allow a free and frank discussion of their tenets and dogmas because most of them lack the grand experience of the founder that brought their faith into existence. If they had it even once, the situation would be quite different and, confident of their own position, for true mystical experience engenders a faith that no fault-finding can shake, they would welcome healthy criticism, and by their very life prove the truth of the basic doctrines of all great religions, lying barren beneath a crumbling mass of superstition and a ponderous load of ceremonies, rituals, and practices, the cobwebs which every prophet, mystic, and seer tried to clear in his time, only to expose his own message to the same process of encrustation soon after his departure from the earth, to become more prolific and tenacious than the one he had swept away.

Those who hold that the founder or founders of their religion, their mystics and saints, had the supreme vision and performed their holy tasks of regenerating mankind as a special prerogative of God, and that they had been sent purposely for the mission assigned to them, do a great injustice not only to the lofty men who, acting as messiahs, tried to elevate mankind by their own example and precept, but also to the Supreme Source of all creation by attributing arbitrariness, partiality, and nepotism to a system of existence bound by law from end to end. The anthropomorphic conception of a God, dealing out favors left and right, watching over the actions of his children like a jealous father, propitiated by acts of remembrance and small offerings and always on the look out to punish those who offend him or forget to pay homage in the prescribed way, cannot but cramp man's

highly developed imagination and constantly rankle his penetrating intellect. We have, therefore, to search for some other explanation than those now offered to account for the inexplicable
phenomena associated with Yoga and mysticism, and for the
appearance from time to time of extraordinary spiritual prodigies, who tried in diverse ways to popularize noble ideals of
love, brotherhood, and peace on the blood-stained arena of the
earth.

There are still some people, though their number is now on
the decrease, who ascribe visionary religious experiences to a
pathological or hysterical condition of the mind. They make no
difference between illuminative states experienced by a contemplative and the delusions of a psychotic. While it must be
admitted that the biological factors which pave the way to
spiritual experience can, in disharmonious states of the body or
mind, or unfavorable heredity, cause pathological affections of
various kinds, it is as fallacious to attribute the phenomenon
of spiritual unfoldment to a morbid state of the mind as it
would be to ascribe the conditions attending pregnancy and
childbirth to an unhealthy state of the body. To stigmatize genuine religious experience as a kind of mania would mean to ascribe some of the loftiest creations of the human mind in the
sphere of literature, art, philosophy, and ethics to the erratic
efforts of a mad man. If we cannot understand the phenomenon
it is not sensible to resort to solutions that savor of sterility. A
far better course would be to make greater efforts to solve the
riddle and to refrain from explanations until our knowledge has
developed sufficiently to make a fruitful investigation possible.
To ignore a factor that has been responsible for half the events
of history and has proved the greatest incentive for human
progress has been a serious omission on the part of those competent to make the investigation. Failure to meet the challenge
of a phenomenon so remarkable, so far-reaching and widespread
in its effects, so intriguing and baffling in its nature as religion
has always proved to be, can mean only one of three things in

the present state of man's progress. Either there is a sense of defeat even before the exploration has been started, or an unaccountable prejudice toward religion and the Divine exists, or the present evolutionary development of the mind tends more toward the material and the gross than toward the spiritual and the sublime.

There is a class of scholars who, though themselves intensely religious and God-fearing, refrain from the inquiry on the plea that the sacramental and the holy should always remain beyond the touch of reason, and that the ways of God and the prophets are not amenable to intellectual investigation. Such an attitude of mind is not one of submission but of antagonism to the laws of God, for if He had decreed that reason should not meddle in the affairs of faith, then religion would have remained confined to the spirit alone and never encroached upon the province of the flesh. But since every prophet and every inspired sage tried to regulate the behavior of the body so as to make mortal life in harmony with spiritual laws, this constitutes an invitation, even a command, to the intellect, which is a part of the body, to aid in making this harmony not only possible but also fruitful. For a number of reasons the modern intellect has shown an apathy toward the investigation of the phenomenon of religion which is completely at variance with the zeal evinced by it in other directions. The upshot has been that many infantile beliefs, dogmas, and practices still continue to obsess the mind of a large proportion of the human race, which is not only incommensurate with their intellectual stature, but also positively dangerous for their survival. The fact that a few intellectuals here and there put forward what appear to be rational interpretations of the religious idea and belief in defense of faith, does not serve to change the general atmosphere of doubt toward the expression of what is one of the fundamental urges of the human mind.

One other explanation that the Yoga trance or mystical experience is the outcome of self-hypnosis and suggestion, though

applicable in a number of cases, does not at all help us to understand genuine spiritual illumination. It can explain the ecstasy,
the visions, and the exaltation, but not the permanent, uplifting
effect of the experience on the whole of life. It cannot explain the
certitude gained of immortality, or the magnetic influence exercised, or the, at times, psychic gifts displayed; and, above all, it
cannot explain the dazzling light of genius shed from ancient
times by some of the brighest stars of this constellation. In the
literature of the world is there anything to compare with the
sublimity of the Upanishads, the Bible, the Quran, the dialogues
of Buddha, and the teachings of the Gita? Does any other work
contain the same inimitable arrangement of words, the same
depth, persuasive power and appeal?

If the answer to this is negative does it not mean that besides
their divine mission these religious preceptors also rank among
the greatest geniuses the earth has ever produced for the literary
excellence of their works? The achievement appears all the more
phenomenal when it is remembered that some of these authors
were illiterate, some imperfectly lettered, and only a few of them
having any pretension to scholarship. Besides them there are
hundreds of comparatively lesser known ecstatics who, circumscribed by the environments in which they were born, shed their
brilliance within the periphery of a small locality, but nonetheless,
within their own province and relating to their own language,
their works possess the same excellence as the more widely known
contributions of the world-renowned founders of great religions
and top-rank illumined seers.

We are, therefore, face to face with a mighty problem when
we try to find an explanation for the mental condition of the
religious teachers of the highest order. We have to account for
the existence of not one but four outstanding attributes of front-
rank mystic minds. They are Ecstasy, Moral Elevation, Psychic
Powers, and Genius. This remarkable combination is confined to
this class, and this class alone. Otherwise we find these attributes
distributed singly and in too few cases. The combination of even

two out of them in one individual is extremely rare. The man of genius may not have moral elevation, ecstatic vision, or psychic gifts, a medium may not have moral stature, vision, or genius, and one prone to visionary states may not have the moral armor, psychic power, or the genius of the true mystic. In judging the prophet, the mystic, and the real saint we have to take the startling fact into consideration that he is in possession of all four rare and lofty attributes, each one of which, even when singly present, confers distinction on one possessing it. There is no difference except one of degree between a genuine prophet, mystic, accomplished Yogi, seer, and sage, and whoever out of them emerged with all these four gems glittering in his crown.

It is obvious that no explanation offered either now or in the past provides a satisfactory solution to the riddle. What makes the phenomenon more inexplicable is the evidence of authentic cases in which the whole gamut of mystical flight of the soul has been experienced by some persons who neither underwent any discipline nor were religious nor even believed in God. For some of them nature assumed the aspect of divinity, and they experienced all the emotions—the sense of awe, enlargement of consciousness, the sense of oneness with creation, overwhelming idea of deathlessness and unlimited knowledge—which are associated with mystical experience. It does not matter whether the ecstasy was repeated frequently or occurred only once or twice, but what is of utmost importance in judging the phenomenon is the inescapable fact that, apart from the category of mystics and Yoga saints, human consciousness shows the capacity of enlargement in the direction of a supersensory, widely extended state, in some persons even without any discipline or training, denoting a potentiality of the human body which the various methods are designed to develop. This clearly points to the existence of a psychic or organic activity in man by which this extraordinary metamorphosis of consciousness is effected.

Commenting on the significance of ecstasy, William James writes: "Saint Ignatius was a mystic, but his mysticism made him assuredly one of the most powerfully practical human engines that ever lived. Saint John of the Cross* writing of the intuitions and 'touches' by which God reaches the substance of the soul, tells us that—'They enrich it marvellously. A single one of them may be sufficient to abolish at a stroke certain imperfections of which the soul during its whole life had vainly tried to rid itself, and to leave it adorned with virtues and loaded with supernatural gifts. A single one of these intoxicating consolations may reward it for all the labours undergone in its life—even were they numberless. Invested with an invincible courage, filled with an impassioned desire to suffer for its God, the soul is then seized with a strange torment—that of not being allowed to suffer enough.' "

Where is this new center of spiritual energy formed? From which mysterious source comes the vision, the celestial joy which, as St. Teresa says, "Penetrates to the very marrow of one's bones," the lucidity that sees to the very foundations of the universe and the sense of unity that merges one with All? Secular knowledge has no answer to this question. "To the medical mind," says William James, "these ecstasies signify nothing but suggested and imitated hypnoid states, on an intellectual basis of superstition, and a corporeal one of degeneration and hysteria. Undoubtedly these pathological conditions have existed in many and possibly in all the cases, but that fact tells us nothing about the value for knowledge of the consciousness which they induce. To pass a spiritual judgment upon these states, we must not content ourselves with superficial medical talk, but inquire into their fruits for life."

But an answer to it is provided in the Tantras, the Upanishads, Sufi literature, the self-revelations of Christian mystics, and the esoteric doctrines of almost all religions both ancient and modern. In fact the whole ponderous superstructure of religion that has been progressively gathering substance from prehistoric times

* *Collected Works,* transtated by Otilio Rodriguez, Doubleday, New York, 1964.

contains the most effective answer to this question. The impulse to find the Creator, the search for magical powers to rise beyond the inexorable laws of the material world, the desire for immortality and the yearning for an ideal state of existence, which have been an inherent feature of the human mind, in crude and nebulous forms in the primitive state, must have a place of origin in the organism of man which not only produced the initial seed but has continued to water the growing plant for the past many thousand years in all the vicissitudes through which mankind has passed.

It is a striking testimony to the anomalous behavior of the human mind that an impulse which received the greatest share of attention from the outstanding intellects during past epochs should, in this age of reason, be the target of a most irrational prejudice which refuses to accord even recognition to it, as a basic urge reaching up from the deepest strata of man's being. Nothing would, perhaps, appear more fantastic to a modern intellectual than to hold that the impulse to reach God or the desire to gain miraculous powers, immortality, or an ideal state of being does not merely rest on fancy or wish-fulfillment or any other imaginary cause, but rather on a solid basis provided for it by nature in mankind. Just as travel at incredible speeds in interplanetary space represents an achievement beyond the wildest dreams of the leading thinkers of the seventeenth or eighteenth centuries, in the same way the discovery of the marvelous Fount of Spiritual Energy, which is at the bottom of all these impulses and desires, would place in the hands of the elite of the coming centuries a veritable mine of new knowledge and possibilities entirely beyond the imagination of the thinkers of our time.

7

The Biological Aspect of *Kundalini*

In general, when discussing religion and the gospels of the various faiths, we are apt to confine our attention to the period, very recent in the annals of man, during which the present well-known religions of mankind have been in existence, and we often entirely overlook the epochs prior to that through which man lived as a rational being, active and alert with crude stone implements to hunt, arboreal shelters, caves, skin tents or hovels, and with but the rudiments of savage culture to regulate his family and social behavior. He continued to live in this manner, split up into various ethnic groups, and scattered over different regions of the earth, at the mercy of the elements, surviving with the greatest difficulty the awful rigor of the glacial periods that covered a large part of the earth for long periods of time. Through this period man was never without a religion, however crude and primitive, but a religion nevertheless. This religion often took revolting and fantastic forms and shapes, sometimes demanded horrible sacrifices and awful austerities, but there was always a religion of some sort to occupy his mind in all the epochs before the birth of existing faiths, varying from place to place and age to age.

Computing roughly, the current faiths, and even those of which some sort of historical record is available, do not extend to more than five or six thousand years, whereas the primitive faiths cover a period of more than five or six times this time. It is true that these faiths were for the most part a jumble of myth, superstition, magical rites, sorcery, blood sacrifices and weird rituals in which our cultured minds can see nothing but dark distortions of the holy and the sacred. Nonetheless these wild and fantastic outpourings were the uncontrolled and unrefined expression of an inner urge that tried to find some sort of meaning in human life, and to make a distinction between the physical and the superphysical parts of man.

Primitive man made a distinction between the visible world and the unseen, between the corporeal body and the spirit, between the waking state and dreams, between here and the hereafter, between the sacred and the profane. He looked at the mysterious forces of nature with awe and an ever-growing desire to come in contact with the powers that controlled these forces, or the spirits that animated them. He ate, drank, frolicked and fought, worked and slept always under the shadow of mysterious powers that surrounded him, brought him abundance and dearth, disease and health, and in other ways ruled his destiny. In one form or another all the characteristics of the religious impulse, and all the symptoms of the inexpressible longing for the supernatural and the supersensible, were present in man in crude and amorphous forms for many many thousands of years before the sages, the saviors, and the prophets came, one after the other, to refine the crude distorted beliefs and to humanize the cruel and revolting rites and practices that had gathered shape in his savage mind through staggering spans of earlier times.

Crude forms of Yoga must have been in use for thousands of years, in almost all parts of the earth, before it took shape as a regular system in India. The problem that now arises is how to account for an impulse seated so deep in human nature that it has persisted through many ages, perhaps even from the first glimmer of reason in man, overpowering his mind to such an extent that it swayed all his actions and thoughts and kept him in thrall from birth to the moment of death, and even pursued him to the hereafter, instilling in him a desire for ceremonial burial and performance of rituals after his death. It certainly could not be a passing fancy or a transient reaction, created in his yet insufficiently developed, ignorant mind, by its first impact with natural phenomena and the effort to find an explanation for them. It could also not be the outcome of fear of the elements in a state of fury, the thunder and lightning, the wind and tide, the rain and storm, since he was accustomed and reconciled to them from the very beginning of his career on earth millions of years before. It is amazing that such lame explanations have been put forward by eminent scholars to rationalize an impulse that has been one of the most powerful governing factors of man's existence from primeval times.

From the unmistakable evidence before us it is obvious that at no time in his checkered career was man free from the mental fervor characteristic of the religious urge. On the contrary, with few exceptions he seems to have been much more in the grip of the supernatural than the most credulous and the most superstitious of today. There is no other single factor, apart from the primary urges, that has maintained such a hold on the mind of primitive man, diverting his activity into channels that had absolutely no relationship with the satisfaction of his physical needs. He could have continued to survive without it, even after the advent of reason, as he had survived for millions of years before in the subhuman and animal stages. Viewed from a strictly rational perspective it can be said that the religious impulse, instead of aiding the development of reason, enveloped the mind with darkest clouds of superstition and fear, and continues to do so even now in the lower strata of underdeveloped societies. But at the same time there is no denying the fact that, side by side with his reason, this mysterious impulse of submission to unseen intelligent forces around him, and a dim sense of the distinction between this world and the other, between the propitious and unpropitious or the holy and the unholy, spontaneously took shape in his mind. This did not disappear with the advance of the intellect, as shadows disappear at the approach of light, but became more rational, keeping the same hold on the seasoned intellect as it had done thousands of years before when reason was still in its infancy.

A few words are necessary to weigh the validity of some of the hypotheses put forward by modern scholars and men of science to account for the phenomenon of religion. One of these, the doctrine of the animistic origin of religion, was propounded by E. B. Taylor, an anthropologist of the nineteenth century, and by Herbert Spencer, a well-known writer on philosophical subjects. According to this theory the investiture by the primitive mind of all the objects and forces of nature with life or animation in the form of soul, spirit, or other invisible beings provides the basis for the appearance of the organized religions of later epochs. The idea of aliveness or animation in nature, it is supposed, originated in the mind of primitive man from the observation of death scenes, when the living principle seems to depart from the body; from dreams, hallucinations, trance conditions, or from what the savage could only interpret as the animated activity of natural forces. This idea, it is held, materialized first in ancestor worship and in funeral rites and ceremonies in the belief that the departed souls or spirits led an invisible existence of their own.

Apart from the fact that the practice of worshiping the spirits of the departed has not been universal, the theory of the animistic origin of religion fails to explain the various amorphous forms of religious motivation exhibited in the still earlier ideas of primitive man, as for instance, in totemic practices or in the notions of mana and taboo. There might have been other variations, too, of which we have no knowledge. So far as the animistic idea is concerned it speaks more in favor of the hypothesis that religion is the expression of a basic impulse of the psyche and from the very beginning started in the human mind as a distinction between the body and the spirit, this world and the other, death and deathlessness, the permissible and unpermissible, the sacred and profane, as a spontaneous projection of an inner development that slowly and painfully, but at the same time inexorably, led evolving mankind to the lofty conceptions that now permeate the religious literature of the world. From a rational point of view, therefore, animism ought to be considered as an inevitable phase in the evolution of the religious impulse, and early mode of its expression, and not as the well-spring of religion itself.

For the hypothesis of the psychoanalytical school, founded by Freud, it is enough to say that the Freudian concept is not now fully accepted by some other psychologists. Another eminent psychologist, McDougall, believes in the existence of an animating principle or soul in the human body. The idea of a Father in heaven, who looks benignly after the created multitudes of humanity and provides for their needs, might well appear to casual observation as the projection of a wish for a protective father, but a deeper study of even such an anthropomorphic concept of God makes this interpretation untenable for the simple reason that the very idea of a superearthly Being, having his abode in high heaven, with divine attributes and able to command all the forces of nature, not being a fact of experience, must depend for its existence on a tendency present in the human mind to draw a distinction between the earthly and the Divine or between this world and the one above or beyond it, and is evidence of the influence of the deep-rooted religious feeling in man. Apart from this, if we cast a glance at the unrefined religious ideas and practices of primitive man we find that this was more often of a compulsive or exacting, than of a pleasure-yielding or wish-fulfilling nature, a driving pressure reaching up from the depths of the primitive mind.

For further clarification it is necessary to point out that at present scholars are practically in the dark as to the nature of psychic energy, the source of all vital activity in the body, including that of thought and the rapid interplay of nerve impulses. No one would like to contend the blatantly obvious fact that thought and consciousness do not fall into the category of material objects according to the current definitions of matter. Yet according to Samkhya-Yoga and Saivite schools of philosophy, the three widely accepted cosmogonic doctrines of Indian thought, dealing with *prakrati*, or matter, as an objective reality (in contrast to Védanta, which treats it as an illusory appearance), not only thought but even the intellect and ego are the manifestations of matter in its ultra-subtle formation.

This classification is based on the introspective study of nervous impulses and analysis of thought in the highly penetrative supersensual states of consciousness or *samadhi*. The scientific value of an exploration carried out in this manner is far greater that that of the somewhat analogous investigation, carried out by men of science, on normal men through an analysis of their dreams, on neurotics and the insane or on hypnotized subjects for the diagnosis of mental and even physical ailments. The amazing knowledge of the nervous system and the flow of two kinds of nerve currents, about which science has no accurate information as yet, has also been obtained in the same manner. The founders of these philosophical schools had a very sound basis for their postulates, for in the superconscious state psychic energy, or *prana,* whether or not brought to a state of arrest, becomes clearly perceptible as an extremely subtle essence in the body, atomic or subatomic in nature, the connecting link between the material organism and immaterial life.

The impossibility of interaction between matter and the incorporeal spirit, without an intermediary connecting link, is an old problem of philosophy. Attempts to meet this difficulty have found an outlet in the various forms of monism, pantheism, Vedanta, and the like. Setting aside the philosophical aspect of the subject, all we wish to emphasize is the fact that the existence of an extremely attenuated biological substance that acts as fuel to the activity of thought and the play of the nervous impulses is a *sine qua non* of biology itself. The present lack of knowledge of this vital biological essence, which is as necessary for the manifestation of life and thought as the fine metal filament in a glass bulb is necessary for the manifestation of electric light, invalidates many of the present-day concepts of psychology based on direct interrelation between the psyche and the physical organism. The moment the existence of this medium is accepted, and, considering the highly sensitive devices that are now coming into use for the measurement of psychic activity, it should not take long to locate it. The present tendency to ascribe almost every obscure phenomenon of the mind, such as neurosis, lunacy, hysteria, ecstasy, dream and religious experiences exclusively to the subconscious must cease to obsess the intellect. In that event it would be saner to infer that the object affected is not the soul, an immaterial, universal substance, which cannot become diseased by material contamination. But it is the interconnecting medium, or *prana* which is the fuel of thought and which when even slightly disturbed or disorganized creates the disintegrations and distortions of personality peculiar to affections of the mind.

The view of Freud that religions originated in some primitive situations in which the sons combined to kill their father that they might possess his wives and concubines, but felt so guilty after the murder that they refrained from such possession, repented for their deeds through religious rites. The inaccuracy of this view is apparent. How could a solitary or even a few incidents of this kind lead to the establishment of a practice and the development of a compulsive need, throughout the primitive world, of such an overwhelming character as to sway the conduct, thought, and history of mankind to this day. Also how could the thought of performing posthumous religious rites, as a measure of repentance, occur to the sons of the murdered father if religion in some form or, at least, the idea of survival of the spirit of the departed was not present in their minds? If the idea was already current at the time it means that religion had originated before the incident.

Another hypothesis for the origin of religion, put forward by

Wilhelm Schmidt, rests on the assumption that originally there was worship of one high or supreme God or a few high gods, which later proliferated into the worship of countless smaller gods, spirits, ghosts or demons among primitive people. The idea of a High God can only spring from the natural tendency in the human mind to seek out the author or cause of every object one confronts. The primitive mind had to follow this tendency in order to postulate a Creator or Father for the existence of the world round it, however crude that conception might have been, and however narrow and limited the cosmos might have appeared to its still imperfectly developed conceptual faculty. Thus there can be no dispute about any hypothesis presented for the existence of an Author or Progenitor of the world. But when it is accompanied by the idea of offering worship to this self-created Progenitor, combined with the concept of His unceasing control over the forces of nature, His incorporeality, omnipotence and immunity to death, the position becomes entirely different. It demands a deeper probing into the human mind, whether primitive or civilized, in order to discover the cause for all the emotional and intellectual ferment associated with religion from the very earliest times.

The idea of Durkheim that totemism was the most primitive and universal form of religion and that as the god of a clan the totemic principle could be nothing else than the clan itself, personified and symbolized, means that it was the society that evoked the experience of the Divine in the mind of primitive man by virtue of the power it had over him. The society required that, forgetful of his own interests, he should make himself its servant and submit to every sort of inconvenience, deprivation and sacrifice without which social life would be impossible. As the social structure of the group is expressed in spiritual ways, the individual came to believe that it was outside or beyond himself. This theory does not explain how the idea of the totem itself originated. Why should the primitive mind have imagined that a certain intimate relationship existed between himself and some animal or plant, or have regarded it as of particular significance for tribe and paid reverence to it? The very fact that an institution of this sort existed in more primitive forms of human society with the rudiments of worship and solemnity attached to it provides ample evidence for the existence of a peculiar impulse in the aboriginal human mind that expressed itself as an invisible relationship between itself and some animal or plant, some object or force in nature. The primitive mind invested it with life and the power to act evilly or benignly toward him, his whole family or clan demanding a reverential and solemn attitude or some sacrifice for its propitiation, with a promise of bestowing strength and power if worshiped with due ceremony. In this way the very existence of totemism denotes the activity of the religious impulse in rudimentary form.

Another school of thought traces the origin of religion to magic. It is, no doubt, a well-observed fact that in one form or another belief in magic has been widespread among primitive people all over the earth. This either took the form of spells or charms or rites performed to influence disembodied spirits, ghosts, demons, and other invisible forces of nature, for gaining the objectives not ordinarily possible, such as curing disease, granting favors, harming an enemy, winning an object of passion, or for other purposes. As in the case of fetishism, the symbol rested on the investiture of some natural object, an image, a pebble, a piece of bone, a feather of a particular bird or any such small thing or article with the power of warding off evil or granting desires. Another form of magic is contained in Shamanism, another very widespread primitive cult in existence even now among the Eskimos of North America, northern Asia and the primitive peoples of the Pacific and African regions. The Shamans, in a state of ecstasy, or possessed by a spirit or some psychic power, exhibit curative, clairvoyant, or magical powers. According to J. G. Frazer, magic is the basic substance out of which religion has probably developed. Where magic failed to achieve the aims desired, the primitive mind, he says, turned to religious practices to attain them.

Magic is the companion and not the precursor of religion. Although it does not now form a part of the modes of worship and the rituals of the major faiths of mankind, it is inherent in their origins and in the lives or teachings of their founders under the guise of the "miraculous." Buddha sternly disallowed the use of psychic powers, but he admitted their existence, and the possibility of their development in one who strives for deeper insights. There is a tradition that he had to demonstrate his own magical powers when for the first time he returned to his own kingdom after enlightenment. The miraculous is no more than divinized magic. The eight *siddhis* or psychic powers, attributed to Yoga, are merely developed forms of magical skill. The magical feats of Shamans are duplicated every day in varied forms by mediums and sensitives of civilized communities. How many religious-minded people offer worship to the Deity purely as a mark of reverence and devotion without any ulterior, temporal or spiritual, objective? For a large part of mankind are not religious observances and prayer a propitiatory approach to Divinity for success in worldly pursuits, freedom from affliction or for the cure of an intractable disease by special favor or, in other words, by a miraculous intervention? There has been no time when religion was free of the magical and the miraculous. Sorcery, witchcraft, necromancy, crystal-gazing, prophecy, and all the other forms of magic-craft and divination originate from the same source in which the religious impulse has its birth.

The unmistakable similarity in the early crude religions, totemic practices and the mana-taboo concepts of primitive peoples, separated by insuperable barriers and unconquerable distances, clearly points to the fact that man's response to an inner motivation has been practically the same, marked by divergences due to varied environments and different mental levels of the tribes. The more elaborate magical practices, religious ideas, and rituals of the vanished civilizations of Sumer, Egypt, Chaldea, Babylon, Crete, and the Indus Valley show another phase in this development. The teachings of the later prophets, saviors, and sages, known to history, demonstrate a further striking advance over the former. But a close observation clearly shows the existence of an unmistakable vein of identity running through them. This is a clear indication of the fact that the development of the religious idea in man has proceeded in a visibly uniform manner from the earliest ages to this day. From this it follows that those adherents of the existing faiths, who hold that the last word on the subject is contained in their gospels, and that man has nothing more to learn about religious truths, adopt an attitude of resistance to the natural evolutionary growth of the religious impulse.

There are also other views about religion. Hegel considers religion to be a permanent and independent activity of the spirit, next in importance to philosophy. According to Kant, religion consists in regarding all our duties as divine commands. Equating of morality with religion does not, however, explain the extremely varied phenomena of the latter. It is true that religion has a close relationship to morality or to what is permissible or not permissible, but the two are not identical. Moreover, what we treat as "divine commands" in the savage cults sometimes assumed the form of horrible human sacrifice, which by no stretch of imagination can be classed as moral, although the attitude of mind that led to those sacrifices and other atrocities was undoubtedly religious. According to the idea of Rudolf Otto, the basis of religion is a feeling for which he has used the word "numinous" —a kind of divine respect distinguishable from mere fear or terror. In its lower form it may be regarded as the feeling excited by the weird and the uncanny. Included in this numinous feeling is the sense of mystery which is never absent from true religion.

Whatever the explanation offered, there can be no two opinions about the fact that this feeling, impulse, or attitude of mind, is not uniformly distributed among individuals, but radically varies in its intensity, from total preoccupation with it, utter neglect of the world, to the seemingly almost complete absence of this feeling. We see both types of people around us. There are those in whom religion assumes the form of a ruling passion, and who do not hesitate to sacrifice everything to satisfy the overmastering impulse in diverse ways, and those whom the idea of the supernatural, the religious or the sacramental leaves entirely unaffected. From the accounts of their lives we are left in no doubt as to the incontestable position that almost all the great saviors, prophets, mystics, and seers were men and women with an overmastering passion for the spiritual and the divine, which often drove them to such heights of sacrifice and suffering, heroic actions and courageous deeds, and to such levels of nobility and benevolence as have few parallels in any other sphere of human activity. Many of them faced death and martyrdom, torture and abuse without flinching or even swerving a step from the path they had chosen for themselves and which, under a direction surpassing mortal will and choice, they believed was chalked out for them by an Almighty Divine Power or Being.

For a proper study of the phenomenon of religion the correct way is not to concentrate only on the gospels, rituals, ceremonies, and their effectiveness as a means to assuage the spiritual thirst of the adherents of one particular faith or of all the modern faiths and creeds, but to focus attention on the mode of expression of the religious impulse from dim antiquity to the present day. In making this study, a fruitful method is to carry out an examination of the mental conditions, behavior, and utterances of the individuals in whom the impulse attained its fullest expression.

At present, unfortunately, the world is sharply divided into two mutually antagonistic strata, one of which, the believers, profess implicit faith in the beliefs and tenets of their religion and the other, the nonbelievers, who deny as uncompromisingly the authenticity and truth of such beliefs. The result is that the whole issue has become controversial where religion is looked upon more as a matter of individual choice and opinion or, in plain language, as a hobby or even a fad, rather than as an indispensable activity of the mind or an innate urge of the human psyche. The devout are as responsible for this as the skeptics, for the simple reason that they surround the founders of their religions or their prophets and sages with such a background of miracles and supernatural occurrences, or such an atmosphere of divinity, that they are elevated to the stature of superhuman beings, completely removed from the sphere of men of flesh and blood. This deification of a specially gifted class of mortals, who are as human as any of us, with the difference that they have an inordinate passion for the Divine and are prone to mystical states that permeate their whole life, and in most cases cause them to renounce all the pleasures of flesh, is causing more damage to religion and to the colossal possibilities it possesses for the unification and regeneration of mankind than all the other factors of human experience.

It is easy to see that not one of the explanations offered, either by men of science or by those of faith, is able to cover all the innumerable facets of the religious phenomenon. Most of the attempts made to present a solution, broadly speaking, fall into two categories. They either display an orchestration of learning which overawes the less learned into an acceptance of the theory merely by an exhibition of erudition or attempt an intellectual investigation on the basis of the data collected, both of them unsatisfactory methods for approaching the numinous. For a real understanding of the problems arising from religion it is necessary that the exponent should have undergone the experience himself. It is a curious fact that while in the allied branches of knowledge, as for instance biology, biochemistry and psychology, empirical study is considered an essential qualification for a writer in these subjects the equally if not more important and more widely sought-after sphere of religion has been left open for the invasion of any charlatan, dabbler, or impersonator, who wishes to make it a hunting ground for his amusement or gain.

We have already arrived at the conclusion that, whatever the explanation offered for the existence of the religious impulse, there can be no doubt about the fact that in those who attained the higher peaks of spiritual ascent, and flowered as inspired prophets and illumined sages, the impulse was invariably strongly marked from the beginning or developed at some period in life.

No mere dabbler and no impostor ever rose to the heights of spiritual glory or ever found a place in the lofty cadre of the illuminati. The utmost that any exceedingly clever imitator or actor ever achieved was the unenviable reputation of a thaumaturgist or a magician. The highest products of spiritual discipline in every part of the earth enjoy a reputation for sanctity and nobility that has been seldom reached by any other class of men.

If a study is made of all the top-rank prophets, mystics, sages, and seers of the earth, whether they were Christians, Muslims, Hindus, Buddhists, Taoists, or Zoroastrians, it will be found that all of them, and they number hundreds, were in possession of all Transcendent attributes in varying proportions. Viewed dispassionately this singular combination of higher mental faculties in religious geniuses is of profound significance and can point to only one momentous conclusion which is that the religious impulse, acting in an inexplicable manner, blossoms ultimately into a personality which, from our generally accepted standards, is of the loftiest stature. This means, in other words, that the religious urge, functioning in a strong, well-marked form, is the harbinger of a higher state of consciousness, mental efficiency, moral enlightenment, and supernormal psychic gifts.

The following passage, from the Foreword to the Introduction to Zen Buddhism, written by Jung, helps to illustrate our meaning: "It could be objected that consciousness in itself has not changed, only the consciousness of something, just as though one had turned over the page of a book and now saw a different picture with the same eyes. I am afraid this is no more than an arbitrary interpretation, for it does not fit the facts. The fact is that in the texts it is not merely a different picture or object that is described, but rather an experience of transformation, often occurring amid the most violent psychic convulsions. The blotting out of one picture and its replacement by another is an everyday occurrence which has none of the attributes of a transformation experience. It is not that something different is seen, but that one sees differently. It is as though the spatial act of seeing were changed by a new dimension. When the Master asks: 'Do you hear the murmuring of the brook?' he obviously means something quite different from ordinary 'hearing.' Consciousness is something like perception, and like the latter is subject to conditions and limitations. You can, for instance, be conscious at various levels, within a narrower or wider field, more on the surface or deeper down. These differences in degree are often differences in kind as well, since they depend on the development of the personality as a whole; that is to say, on the nature of the perceiving subject."

Jung's own solution of the problem does not explain the reason for the transformation of consciousness, which he admits. For every manifestation of the phenomenon of religion he ultimately turns to the Unconscious, a self-invented magic key which with a little verbal turning and twisting, can be made to fit into any lock. The transformation of consciousness does not, in the genuine cases, point to a subconscious content of the mind nor to the collective unconscious, from the primeval savage to the modern intellectual, but to a state of awareness which, transcending the limits of time and space, can exercise the faculties of enhanced knowledge, clairvoyance, and prophetic vision for which psychology has no explanation to offer at all. This metamorphosis of consciousness is not of the nature of a subjective experience only, but coming with enhanced intellectual efficiency, supernormal psychic gifts, and moral elevation provides conclusive evidence of the fact that the change has affected the very roots of being, and shows a difference of the same kind as is present between a man of mediocre mental ability and an intellectual prodigy. When we never allow ourselves to remain in doubt about the fact that there must exist a biological distinction between the former type of mind and the latter, it is really strange that we fail to allow the same difference between the common run of human beings and the illuminati.

In the absence of a satisfactory explanation from any modern source we are driven to look into the ancient volumes relating to the subject for a solution of the problem. When we do so we find that the phenomenon of transformation, transfiguration, conversion, transmutation, or rebirth is fully recognized by almost all the religions and occult doctrines of the past. While every faith and occult creed possesses its own method of physical and mental training to effectuate this transformation there is no unanimity among them either about the nature of the transformation effectuated or the factors responsible for it. At the present moment hardly anyone is prepared to acknowledge that there is a regular psychosomatic arrangement in the body by which approach to Divinity and higher planes of consciousness becomes possible. For the scholar as well as for the common man, religious experience is a subjective phenomenon, although its effects may give rise to objective results. In this context the remarks of William James* are of particular interest: "When, however, a positive intellectual content is associated with a faith-state, it gets invincibly stamped in upon belief, and this explains the passionate loyalty of religious persons everywhere to the minutest details of their so widely differing creeds. Taking creeds and faith-state together, as forming 'religions,' and treating these as purely subjective phenomena, without regard to the question of their 'truth' we are obliged, on account of their extraordinary influence upon action and endurance, to class them amongst the most important biological functions of mankind. Their stimulant and anaesthetic effect is so great that Professor Leuba, in a recent article, goes so far as to say that so long as men can use their God, they care very little who he is, or even whether he is at all. 'The truth of the matter can be put,' says Leuba, 'in this way: God is not known, he is not understood; he is used—sometimes as meat-purveyor, sometimes as moral support, sometimes as friend, sometimes as an object of love. If he proves himself useful, the religious consciousness asks for no more than that. Does God really exist? How does he exist? What is he? Not God, but life, more life, a larger, richer, more satisfying life, is, in the last analysis, the end of religion.

* Longmans Green, New York, 1903.

The love of life, at any and every level of development, is the religious impulse. At this purely subjective rating, therefore, religion must be considered vindicated in a certain way from the attacks of her critics. It would seem that it cannot be a mere anachronism and survival, but must exert a permanent function, whether it be with or without intellectual content, and whether it be true or false."

It is not God who is used by men but, in actual fact, it is God who is using mortals for a divine purpose which He alone knows. Do we know why we lean so heavily on the Supreme Being who is the cause of our existence? Do we know why we exist at all? If not, our attitude to the still unfathomed mystery of creation should be more reverent and more in keeping with our stature as rational beings. It is the upward pull from Universal Consciousness, or call it God, exerted through the psychosomatic channel of *kundalini,* which is at the bottom of this attitude of reliance on God displayed by the religious-minded of all denominations. What our minds habitually reflect must have its source in the invisible Fount from which all our healthy instincts originate. This is the reason for the idea often expressed by mystics of all countries that God reciprocates in a larger measure the love of His devotees and is always at least as eager to receive the love-sick soul into His arms as the soul is to reach Him. The very existence of the idea of God and its close interconnection with the manifold hopes and fears of the human mind provides in itself a strong testimony in support of the stand that religion is inseparably connected with the whole biological and mental structure of man.

The success of surgical operations and medicines in the treatment of diseases depends entirely on the inherent tendency, present in the living flesh, to fill up and heal the wounds, and to react to the chemical agents that enter into the stomach or the bloodstream. If this tendency did not exist it would be dangerous, even fatal, to perform surgical operations, and medicines would prove of no avail in the treatment of illness. The same law must be operative with varying degrees of effectiveness at the bottom of all religious and occult practices, which means, in other words, that unless there exists a possibility in the body to respond spontaneously to such efforts to create the mental and physiological condition necessary for religious experience no amount of hard work done to achieve success in the enterprise can ever be actualized in the smallest degree. The body and mind are so closely interrelated that a change in one is directly or indirectly reflected in the other. Therefore, any exercises or practices undertaken for causing any kind of change in the mind, as for instance inducing *samadhi* or attainment of paranormal faculties, cannot but have a corresponding effect on the body. To deny that the human body is an indispensable factor in the development of a higher state of consciousness or for the exhibition of supernormal faculties amounts to a negation of the objective reality of the phenomena.

Those who believe in religion and the validity of religious experience must also believe in the capacity of the human body to exhibit the phenomena either as a characteristic present from birth or as a hidden potentiality that can be developed with exercise, or that may spontaneously declare itself at some later period in life—in all the three cases manifested in a manner for which we have no rational explanation at present. If for the expression of normal human consciousness a delicately adjusted intricate biological apparatus is absolutely necessary, how can this unalterable condition be dispensed with for the even higher manifestation of Superconsciousness. We do not think in these terms because we are accustomed to treating the normal human body and normal human consciousness as the last achievement of evolution or created by God, a most erroneous notion stemming from self-conceit. Those who do not believe in religion can dismiss the whole subject as pure fabrication of superstitious minds, as a creation of priests or on any other ground. But those who believe cannot escape the responsibility of finding a rational basis for their faith. They cannot say that religious experience is a random or erratic phenomenon, possible only for some people purely by divine favor or as a peculiarity present in their minds, without any relation whatsoever to the biological construction of their bodies, a by-product of the human psyche, active as a matter of accident, and not as an inherent tendency of every mind.

It is as correct to say that religious striving and occult practices somehow create a particular condition of the mind in which mystical experiences become possible without affecting the body, as it would be to hold that self-mortification helps in causing visionary states in ascetics as it is pleasing to God. These explanations do not help to solve the riddle but, on the other hand, make it more complicated and difficult. How can spiritual exercises change the normal behavior of the mind and make it capable of exhibiting entirely inexplicable paranormal phenomena, and, at the same time, why should asceticism be a feature of the religious impulse, effective to such a degree as to create sometimes an awful thirst for self-torture and self-denial? It is the height of folly in such an important issue to explain one enigma in terms of another, thus creating a vicious circle that can never lead to the heart of the problem. It is because we are often accustomed to regard the religion in which we are brought up merely as a legacy of a prophet or a sage or a line of prophets or sages, rather than as an inherent thirst of the human mind, dependent for its existence on the biological makeup of the organism in the same way as other basic urges exist that we deplorably fail in tracing the origin of all phenomena connected with religion to their real source, and leap from one wrong supposition to the other without arriving at the right solution of the problem.

If we believe in the efficacy of Yoga or other systems of discipline designed to lead to transcendent conditions of consciousness and psychic insights, we will have to accept the existence of a responsive element in the body which is affected by these exercises in such a way as to lead to the development or emergence of new faculties and extraordinary mental states in the organism.

This element can take the form either of a general tendency in the body, a predisposition present in the cerebro-spinal system or of a regular mechanism designed by nature to lead the human mind to higher states of consciousness by its own normal activity or by stimulation through some kind of mental and physical exercise. Neither the religious impulse nor the phenomenon of transcendence to which it leads in rare cases can be purely psychic in origin, for in that case, apart from the fact that there can be no uniformity in its manifestation, there would arise no need for somatic disciplines to develop it. There can be no rational explanation of religious and supernormal psychic phenomena other than that there does exist an agency in the mind-body combination which is at the back of the religious impulses and all the consequences that flow out from it. There is no other way to account for the extraordinary happenings of history caused by the impact of illumined men and women, who time after time changed the course of the lives and thoughts of millions of men, and even now continue to exert a tremendous influence in shaping the history of the modern world.

Yoga or any other system of spiritual discipline can, when successful, lead to higher states, or, we can even say, to normally inaccessible levels of consciousness, not by any unnatural methods causing arrest of thought or respiration, as is sometimes supposed, but by a hitherto unthought-of transformation of the human brain. This transformation occurs by means of a mechanism already present in the body. In the initial stages, or where a permanent transformation is not possible, there may occur transient interludes of lucidity or superconsciousness, known as *samadhi,* in the case of Yogis and ecstasy or rapture in the case of mystics. Permanent transformation results in a Jiwan Mukhta, Cosmic-Conscious Yogi, or in an illumined sage. In every case the transformation depends on the awakening of *kundalini.* Protracted practice of meditation and *pranayama* in a determined Sadhaka may lead to the awakening of the serpent power in a few cases. In other cases either a comatose condition, resembling

animals in a state of hibernation, with nearly suspended animation and insensibility or self-induced hypnosis, with highly attenuated breathing, numbness of the body and hallucinatory
experiences, may crown the laborious efforts of some of the practitioners out of the thousands who undertake the discipline. The
rest remain barren of any appreciable results. The awakening of
the serpent power by even the most strenuous Hatha-Yoga
methods is a rare occurrence, and rarer still is its ascent to
sahasrara and its permanent abode in this region, when only the
transformation of the brain is accomplished and Cosmic Consciousness attained.

The spinal cord, with the reproductive equipment at one end
and the ventricular cavity in the brain at the other, is the largest
repository of the life force, or *prana,* in the human body. This
life force is a biochemical substance of a most complex formation,
extremely subtle and volatile, having its roots probably in the
subatomic levels of matter. Belief in the efficacy of Yoga as a
time-honored method of self-realization *ipso facto* means belief
in *prana,* for the whole science of Yoga is built on the possibility
of employing *prana* as an instrument for effecting a metamorphosis of the brain and raising it to higher levels of perception.
In every form of Yoga, with a meditative technique or discipline
of the breath, the first object intended to be influenced is *prana.*
The fact that physiologists have no knowledge of this medium
is of no consequence, for up to very recent times there was no
knowledge of vitamins either. If science has not yet been able to
fashion instruments delicate enough to detect this extremely
subtle essence, it does not mean that it does not exist. Yogis have
differed among themselves about the utility of the various methods employed to gain transcendent knowledge about the nature
of the Ultimate Reality, but there is no dispute among them
about the reality of *prana* as the sole agent responsible for success
in any enterprise undertaken to gain higher states of consciousness. From the time of the Vedas to the present day, a long period
of nearly four thousand years, the existence of *prana* as a work-
able instrument of salvation has been accepted by generation

after generation of Yogis and occultists of India, and their combined testimony carries a weight that cannot be lightly brushed aside.

The manner in which the cerebro-spinal system, with the reproductive organs at the lower end, functions as the evolutionary mechanism is one of the most remarkable instances of the ingenuity and economy of nature. The vast network of nerves covering the whole body, penetrating to every hair and pore of the skin, to every cell of the flesh and bones, to every fiber of the muscles and to the tiniest fragment of every internal and external organ, in addition to discharging its highly complex normal function as the communication system of the body, performs also the supreme task of initiating and carrying into effect the evolutionary impulses that have been instrumental in raising man to his present intellectual stature, and are even now at work to mold his brain toward a higher state of cognition or, in other words, to a transcendent state of consciousness. The method by which this is effected, like all other devices of nature, is extremely simple when it is once thoroughly understood. But as long as it is not understood, like other still hidden secrets of existence, it appears so baffling and complicated as to be almost beyond comprehension. The aim of this writing is to draw attention to this amazing but, at the same time, hitherto entirely unsuspected activity of the nervous system. What we have recorded is based word for word on accurately observed personal experience, combined with unmistakable objective proofs, which shall be mentioned at their proper place in another volume. This is not all. Our experience is supported not only by the revelations contained in the vast mass of ancient literature on *kundalini* in Tantras, Manuals on Hatha-Yoga, Upanishads, Puranas, Buddhist documents, and other sacred lore of India, but also by the life stories and utterances of scores of well-known Yoga saints who flourished at various times during the last more than one thousand years and are, therefore, recent figures of history.

Described in terms of modern physiology the activity of the nervous system, in the evolutionary as well as in the reproductive sphere, lies in extracting from the mass of tissue surrounding every nerve fiber an extremely subtle but highly potent essence that may be well designated as concentrated life force, which, traveling along the routes described by the innumerable nerve filaments, ultimately reaches the spinal cord, and the brain, the well-protected storage plants of this highly complex substance. A fraction of it spills over into the nerve junctions and plexuses as also into the nerve clusters lining the various organs. In the case of normal men and women a fine stream of this vital essence trickles through the nerves into the reproductive organs, where it vivifies the sex cells produced by the gonads. It is the existence of this concentrated nerve essence in the spermatozoon and the ovum that bestows fertility and the power of transmission of hereditary characteristics through the genes. The essence permeates every atom of the reproductive cells.

From the upper ending of the spinal cord another fine stream of this living energy filters into the brain as fuel for the evolutionary process continuously at work in the organism. Variations in the size of this stream determine the intellectual and aesthetic development of an individual. The stream is comparatively larger in the case of men of genius and top-rank intellectuals. The variegated expression of genius depends on the particular region of the brain which the cranial stream irrigates and develops. In the accomplished Yogi the nervous system functions in a manner that almost all the subtle *prana,* extracted by the nerves, a large part whereof was formerly expended in procreative activity, now irradiates the brain, resulting in the transformation of consciousness. The whole body, including all the vital organs, participates in this activity of the nervous system in the case of an adept in whom *kundalini* makes her permanent abode in the *sahasrara.* In the case of those in whom ecstasy is experienced at intervals with or without entrancement, this extraordinary activity of the nervous system occurs only for a limited duration at intervals leading to the emergence of a higher consciousness for the time being.

8

The Physiology of Yoga

Before proceeding to describe the mode of operation of the divine Energy, *kundalini,* and the methods devised from ancient times to arouse it to activity, it is necessary to enter into a brief discussion about one point. If *kundalini* is the only natural device in human beings, implanted by nature to lead to transcendent states of consciousness, how has it been possible for the followers of other schools of Yoga and the adherents of other religions to attain the mystical state without awakening this power, and even without having the knowledge that such a force exists designed to stimulate it? Furthermore, if there exists a power center of this kind at all in the human frame, how has it escaped the notice of modern anatomists who have probed into every nook and corner of the body and why when special methods are available to activate it, is the knowledge of the mechanism so rare, even in India, and the number of successful initiates so extremely small as to be almost negligible? There is another important point also: Since *kundalini* is the ultimate source of all the phenomena proceeding from any type of Yoga or any kind of spiritual discipline, how is it that even accomplished Yogis, who achieved transcendence by means of Raja-Yoga, Bakhti-Yoga or Karma-Yoga, or mystics have not been able to detect and locate this hidden power center as Hatha-Yogis and Tantrics have done?

These points are very relevant to the issue and they indirectly support our hypothesis. We have already arrived at the conclusion that religion, in order to be an inherent attribute of the human mind, and not merely an artificial creation of prophets and sages, must have an independent base in the psychic makeup of man, necessitating a complementary biological apparatus as well. The only way by which this psychosomatic contrivance can make its presence felt is to create an awareness in the surface consciousness of the purpose it has to accomplish. This awareness in the initial stages can only take the form of an unaccountable impulse or desire tending, often erratically, in the direction which it is designed to take, like the indefinable sexual propensities of children before they begin to understand the significance of the urge. We have seen how the impulse started in primitive man with the ideas of totem, taboo, death and birth rituals, animism, supernaturalism, and the like, and developed to the point of the worship of spirits, ghosts, living creatures, or natural objects of various kinds and thence rose to the adoration of supernatural entities, celestial beings, gods and goddesses, or one All-pervading God.

During this process of evolution that took man aeons to accomplish there must have been born, at one time or another, peculiarly constituted men and women of the same category, whom we now consider to be mystics, mediums, and sensitives, possessed of unaccountable psychic gifts, but in other respects conforming to the same level of mental development as others. Those of them who were a little more intelligent and tactful than the rest, counting on the awe and wonder they created, must have occupied commanding positions as did the prophets of antiquity, and from that state of authority prescribed, to satisfy the curious crowd, some methods and ways to attain the same powers as they themselves possessed. The appearance of these uncommonly gifted men from the earliest epochs of man's existence should not be in the least surprising. On the contrary it can be taken to be perfectly in accord with the natural order of things. Just as there existed variations in the mental level, physical development and the emotional content of the various people, as is the case even today, there must have also cropped up now and then some odd individuals possessed of uncanny powers, like the medicine-man we even now see among the so-called underdeveloped people, still adhering to religious customs and rituals in vogue thousands of years ago. Their later prototypes still survive in the form of Shamans, voodooists, witchdoctors, and others among the existing primitive societies of the earth.

The inexplicable appearance of mediumistic properties in some persons—telepathy, clairvoyance, divination, and other psychic gifts—cannot be attributed to mere accident, since the attributes are so well defined and the phenomenon has occurred so persistently from earliest time that it would be entirely irrational to ascribe it to the freakish sport of chance. Eliminating chance, the only other rational way to account for it is to accept the possibility of such talent in the psychic endowment of man, about which we are still in the dark, and which is naturally manifest only in an extremely small percentage of people even in this age. This logical conclusion again points to a still obscure activity of the human brain, and the existence of a special region or a center of psychic energy that gives rise to it, in other words, to *kundalini*. These born psychics, part and parcel of the human society from the beginning, are in all probability the instruments designed by nature not only to create interest in the occult and the supernatural, but also to revive interest with their amazing performances whenever it threatens to diminish. It is probably this class of men to which Patanjali refers in his Yoga-Sutras as possessing *siddhis* from birth. By acting on the already present religious impulse in the people of the time, they must have been responsible for the creation of that burning enthusiasm and even frenzy that usually marked the religious zeal of primitive man. In the later epochs this enthusiasm, milder and more refined, was kindled by the oracle and the seer, the more evolved prototypes of the primitive awkward, but still incomprehensible, psychics, known under the names of medicine-men, witchdoctors, Shamans, and the like. Even in this age of reason they are the objects of deep interest for countless millions of people in both the East and the West who are irresistibly drawn to them to assuage their own thirst for the unseen and the supernatural.

The positions of power commanded by these primitive knowers of the occult, as well as their own inherent curiosity and interest, must have acted as a powerful incentive to enterprising individuals, as they do even now, to learn the secrets of the art in order to reach the same position as well as to appease their own thirst for knowledge of supernatural forces with the added motive to harness them to their own service. This must have led to a search for methods and practices to induce the same conditions of mind naturally present in the psychics, and in this search the latter must have played the role of teachers, not always honest ones, to maintain their own position and prestige, which ultimately resulted in the strange practices, orgiastic rituals, hard penances, bloody sacrifices, and bizarre ways of worship that characterized the religious observances of primitive man. Their brutal aspect was in accord with the pattern of his behavior and the level of his mental development. It could not be otherwise, since it would have been entirely unnatural had primitive man been an angel in one respect and a devil in another.

This accumulated store of rites, practices, and exercises, pruned and refined from time to time through the ages, altered and changed by contact with other people and tribes, or revised later by specially gifted magi, oracles or priests, continued to be in the possession of mankind in different parts of the world until, with the further advance of civilization, the practices were again modified and refined by the prophets, sages, and seers, who began to replace the magi, the oracle, the Shaman, the medicine-man and the witchdoctor of primitive peoples. Among the people segregated by sea, deserts, or other natural barriers, the old methods and practices continued to survive until recent times.

As all these methods and practices came into existence as a result of the operation of a naturally active *kundalini* through the ages, and as they were improved and revised from time to time by those in whom the power was naturally awake or was developed in rudimentary forms, it is in keeping with our concept that even without any knowledge of *kundalini,* or any inkling of the practices of Hatha-Yoga, the adherents of other faiths and the followers of other schools of Yoga achieved success with these methods in a limited number of cases. The parent of all systems of religious discipline and ritual from the very beginning of the religions impulse has been *kundalini* alone, and no other agency, human or divine has evoked this impulse.

As regards the other point it is enough to say that there is no separate organ in the body that acts as an evolutionary mechanism for the manifestations associated with *kundalini.* The function is performed by the cerebro-spinal system as a whole through the direct agency of the reproduction mechanism at the base and a still unidentified, silent center in the brain, designated by Indian Savants as *Brahma-rendra* or the Cavity of *Brahma,* which becomes active on the awakening of *kundalini,* resulting in an altered activity of the nervous system. This activity can be verified and measured with proper methods devised for the purpose when the nature of the alteration is understood. It is sufficient to say that the location of this extremely sensitive zone, and the extraordinary sensations to which it gives rise, have been described in precise terms by some of the great mystics and Yoga saints of India. In fact, the paramount importance of this region in every kind of Yoga and every form of meditative technique is universally recognized among all the schools of religious discipline and esoteric practice in India, and finds repeated mention not only in the ancient scriptures and Yoga texts, but in the folklore to such an extent that the close association of this region with success in any form of religious effort is almost as well known as other common concepts of religion.

Like the first whitening of the sky at dawn to herald the approach of the sun, the first sign of success in any form of religious striving comes from this region. It is the place of conjunction of the canal coming from the spinal cord and the ventricles of the brain. This cavity and those adjoining it are filled with the cerebro-spinal fluid, said to be a derivative from the blood and fairly akin to plasma. The whole vast structure of Kundalini-Yoga revolves round this cavity and the spinal canal. For those unacquainted with human anatomy it is only possible to indicate the approximate location of the area on the basis of an inner perception of the region or the sensations experienced there. This, to the best of our knowledge, has also been the means of observation of the ancient masters of this Yoga, which accounts for the variation found in the number of the *nadis* and the *cakras,* and also in their location. It is for this reason that accurate observation and study by experts is necessary in order to place the subject on the footing of an exact science. The effects produced by an awakened *kundalini* are so multilateral from the very beginning to the final stage that once a thorough investigation is started a host of possibilities will come into view, one after the other, by which the biological nature of the phenomenon, from radical changes in the behavior of genital organs to alterations in the activity of the nervous system and the brain can be indisputably established. There is no method so adequate to demonstrate the objective reality of religious phenomena as an investigation carried out on *kundalini.*

The view expressed by Arthur Avalon in his fine book, *The Serpent Power* that the ascent of *kundalini* is always attended by a coldness of the body is applicable only to a very limited number of cases and is not a general characteristic of the awakening. He says: "Kundalini when aroused is felt as intense heat. As Kundalini ascends, the lower limbs become as inert and cold as a corpse; so also does every part of the body when She has passed through and leaves it. This is due to the fact that She as the Power which supports the body as an organic whole is leaving Her center. On the contrary, the upper part of the head becomes 'lustrous,' by which is not meant any external lustre (Prabha), but brightness, warmth and animation. When the Yoga is complete, the Yogi sits rigid in the posture selected, and the only trace of warmth to be found in the whole body is at the crown of the head, where the Shakti is united with Shiva. Those, therefore, who are sceptical can easily verify some of the facts should they be fortunate enough to find a successful Yogi who will let them see him at work. They may observe his ecstasy and the coldness of the body, which is not present in the case of what is called the Dhyana-Yogi, or a Yogi operating by meditating only, and not rousing Kundalini. This cold is an external and easily perceptible sign."

A normal awakening does not arouse intense heat. There is only a pleasant sensation of warmth, beginning from the *muladhara* and spreading to the whole of the body, in the first stages of the Awakening. It is universally accepted by the ancient writers that "heat" resides in the umblical center to carry out the function of digestion. It is, therefore, in accord with this idea to say that *kundalini* burns in the navel. There is also nothing unusual in the expression that the awakening of the serpent power in the umbilical region is revealed by the sensation of a great fire. In fact the ascent of *kundalini* is like the pouring of liquid flame into the various *cakras* and finally into the cranium. It may also resemble the brilliant luster shed by a prolonged flash of lightning, accompanied by noises like thunder. But whether compared to a blazing fire, or flame, or lightning, the idea of intense or burning heat is not included in the expressions for that would introduce an ominous feature into the phenomenon. The repeated mention of the moon in the *sahasrara* and her cool, refreshing luster, made in the ancient works on Kundalini-Yoga, provides ample evidence for our position.

There is no doubt that moderate heat, causing the body to sweat, is caused by *pranayama*, but it is of the same type as is generated by any violent exercise. The word *tapas* used from the Vedic times connotes religious fervor associated with devout worship, self-discipline, and penance, and not to any so-called "mystical heat." *Siddhis* and divine manifestations proceed from *tapas,* as mentioned often in the scriptures. For this reason the only sense in which *tapas* can be understood is intense spiritual effort and austerity and not in the sense of heat, mystical or otherwise. It is often the tendency to find hidden or cryptic meanings in plain words and expressions used by the old authors which cause confusion in the understanding of the phenomena associated with religion and the occult. The expressions "mystic psychic fire-force" and "the Secret Psychic-Heat is born" used in the subjoined passage from the book, *Tibetan Yoga and Secret Doctrines* by W. Y. Evans-Wentz, do not refer to any burning heat, as is also clear from the other passages in the book, but rather to the simple phenomenon of the Awakening, which is here attributed to the transmutation of the seminal fluid. This is explained by Evans-Wentz himself when he says: "Bodhistattvic mind is an honorific term for the male generative fluid or 'moon-fluid.' In the present context it is symbolical of the transmuted sex-vitality, whereby the psychic-heat is produced as are all occult psychophysical powers." It is in this sense that the aforementioned passage, quoted below, is to be understood:

"This is the Tibetan letter-symbol for the personal pronoun 'I' written, $\overset{\circ}{\zeta}$, transliterated as HAM and pronounced as HUM. It is white in correspondence with the sexual fluid, which its visualization sets into psychic activity. The brain psychic-center is conceived as the place whence sexual functions are directed; and, therefore, the HAM is to be visualized as in the chakra called the Sahasrara-Padma, or Thousand-Petalled Lotus. The HAM symbolizes the masculine aspect of the mystic psychic fire-force; and, as a result of its union with that of the feminine aspect, symbolized by the short A, the Secret Psychic-Heat is born. The Goddess Kundalini is roused from her age-long slumber to ascend to her Lord in the pericarp of the Thousand-Petalled Lotus. She first ascends, like a flame, to the Manipura-Chakra, of which the navel is the hub; and the lower half of the body is filled with the mystic fire. Thence she continues her ascent; and in union with her Lord, the Divine One, the whole body is filled, even to the tips of the fingers and toes, with the Secret Psychic-Heat."

The glowing radiance in the head and the light circulating through the nerves gives to the Sadhaka the vivid impression of an inner conflagration, not attended by heat, or of an internal effulgence which fills his whole mental horizon and seems to surround him in and out like a vast circle of flame. Gunjari-pada, quoted by Eliade, also says: "Neither scorching heat nor smoke is found." In the light of this fact it is easy to understand why the ancient savants, in the internal phenomenology, refer to it as the play of fire and compare it to intensely bright objects or heavenly orbs. There is, however, no doubt that in all cases of a healthy Awakening the digestive power is highly augmented. The ancient authors refer to it as increase in the digestive heat: "(with proficiency gained in Pranayama) The digestive-fire (Jathar-Agni) of the Sadhaka is highly increased" "All his limbs become graceful," says Shiv-Samhita (3. 34), "and he partakes of delectable, wholesome foods with great enjoyment. Overflowing with strength and energy his heart is always brimful of joy. (All) these qualities necessarily manifest themselves in the body of the Yogi." Burning heat is created in the body when the *prana* energy, released by *kundalini,* instead of rising through *susumna,* its natural channel, streams partly or wholly through *pingala* or the solar *nadi* on the right side of the spinal cord. It is by arousing the serpent power through the solar nerve that the extraordinary feats of staying naked under ice for prolonged periods or drying wet sheets of linen, wrapped round one's bare body, in Arctic cold can become possible.

The phenomenon of *kundalini* is fraught with so many possibilities that volumes will be required for a detailed treatment of all of them. For our purpose here it is enough to state that the awakening can occur through *ida* or *pingala,* instead of through *susumna,* or partly through one of the former and *su-*

sumna. Where this occurs spontaneously in a forceful manner gravest danger threatens the life and sanity of the unfortunate man or woman. This, so far little understood, morbid awakening of *kundalini* is the root cause of several forms of insanity about which psychiatrists are still groping in the dark. In those in whom the cerebro-spinal system has attained the required degree of maturity the powerful psychic energy set free by *kundalini* invariably makes its abode in the head, raising the consciousness to transcendent planes. Any attempt made by such practitioners to divert the divine energy to this or that nerve channel or this or that *cakra* is fraught with grave danger. In the case of less developed Sadhakas, the force can be raised through *ida* or *pingala* for the performance of a few amazing feats at the cost of the performer's own spiritual welfare and happiness. As *kundalini* is the base of all Yoga practices, the extreme need for caution on the part of those who take to these practices haphazardly, without thoroughly informing themselves about the subject, cannot be overemphasized.

Coming now to our point: the spinal cord, which plays a most important role in the attainment of higher states of consciousness, is a longish white cylinder, oval in cross-section, with an inner gray and outer white matter. Unlike it, the cerebellum and the cerebral hemispheres of the brain have an internal bulk of white and an outer thin layer of gray matter on their surfaces. The cord is encased by the vertebrae, which form a strong bony covering around it. The vertebral column in man consists of thirty-three vertebrae, which fit into one another giving flexibility to the backbone. The direction to sit erect during the course of meditation in Yoga practices is designed to avoid curvature of the cord and the central duct, in which new processes occur and new forces are generated as a result of the pressure exerted on the brain and the nerves by fixity of attention and *pranayama*. In human beings the spinal cord does not extend the whole length of the spinal column, but ends at about the second lumber vertebra, that is, the second vertebra below the thoracic region. In animals with tails (cow, horse, etc.), the spinal cord extends virtually the whole length of the vertebral column. The spinal canal in man does not, therefore, extend to the base of the spine but ends at a point higher up. At the terminus of the spinal cord a cluster of nerves descends below, resembling a horse's tail in appearance, to which the name *cauda equina* has been given.

Thirty-one pairs of spinal nerves arise from the spinal cord, each pair arising in one spinal segment. These segments are not distinguishable internally. Each spinal nerve arises from the cord in two bundles: the dorsal and ventral roots. It is held that the dorsal roots contain afferent, or sensory, nerve fibers, and the ventral roots efferent, or motor, fibers. Along either side of the spinal cord is a chain of ganglia, called the sympathetic chain. These ganglia are connected to another chain of ganglia in front of the vertebral column, which gives rise to the sympathetic plexuses, known as prevertebral ganglia. The third set of sympathetic ganglia situated in the organs is called terminal ganglia. These three sets of ganglia are interconnected among themselves and also with the spinal nerves. Alongside the sympathetic plexuses there is another system of nerves known as the parasympathetic system. Both the sympathetic and the parasympathetic nerves constitute the autonomic nervous system. The most important of the parasympathetic nerves is the vagus, or wandering, nerve, arising from the brain, and passing on the left and right of the spinal column. Most of the visceral organs receive a double innervation, that is both the sympathetic and parasympathetic systems send their nerves to them. In general the fibers from each of these two systems have antagonistic actions on the various organs, which they innervate.

The sympathetic impulses accelerate the heart action and the parasympathetic slow it down. The motility and secretion of the digestive tract are increased by impulses from the parasympathetic nerves, and reduced by sympathetic ones. The same is true of other organs. This augmentative and inhibitory or excitatory and depressive action of the autonomic nervous system has been indicated by the ancient exponents of Hatha-Yoga by the terms *hot* and *cold.* Thus *pingala,* or the solar *nadi,* on the right side of the spinal cord, which rising from the *muladhara cakra* and after criss-crossing with the *ida* at the sites of the various *cakras,* is said to be hot, and *ida,* the lunar *nadi,* on the left side of the spinal canal, which rising from the same place and criss-crossing in the same manner, is said to be cold .The two *nadis* are designated as sun and moon to signify their hot and cold effects. The descriptions of the ancient masters about anatomical and physiological details need not to be taken too literally for the reasons, first, that their knowledge was drawn from subjective experience and not from actual anatomical study and, second, because it was the tendency of the times to clothe physiological knowledge and for that matter knowledge of other natural sciences in metaphoric language, since empirical methods of observation were still in an incipient stage. This holds true not only of Yoga but also of sciences like therapeutics, astronomy, and chemistry, as is obvious from the treatises on these subjects written at that time.

Our task will become easier if for a moment we divest ourselves of the illusion that the ancient writers on the subject were infallible, and deal with Yoga, occult literature, and mystical experience in the same manner, as the first empiricists dealt with the vast store of amorphous theoretical material, dating from very ancient times. Alchemy, astronomy, geography, medicine, biology, and other natural sciences that came to them as a legacy from the past were treated in this way. A reluctance to study empirically religious phenomena can only tend to discredit religion in the eyes of those with a scientific bent of mind, and to create doubt and antagonism against a basic reality and a basic hunger of the human mind. If religious truths are not demonstrable and must always be accepted on faith it means perpetuation of the existing conflicts between the men of faith and the men of science, between religion and religion, creed and creed, and a perpetuaation of doubts and uncertainties. But if they are demonstrable, in order to be lasting, that demonstration should be as possible now as at any time in the future.

Instead of entering into hair-splitting discussions, the wiser

course at the present stage of our knowledge is to concentrate on
the essentials and to find a way out of the labyrinth by treating
only those facts that possess some probability and are not difficult
to fit into the modern concepts of anatomy and psychology. In
order to conform to this mode of presentation it would be necessary to avoid many of the time-honored technical terms and
expressions employed by writers on this form of Yoga, reducing
it to the position of a sectarian cult, and to clothe it in a language
more suited to the rationalistic tendencies of our age and in keeping with the universal nature of the subject itself. Unless we take
the untenable position that for the expression of higher states
of consciousness the human body and the brain need not come
into the picture at all, and that superconsciousness can be achieved
by a sudden plunge into the Unknown, it becomes necessary to
leave no possibility unexplored in order to find some sort of
agreement between the assertions of the ancient authors, writing
under great handicaps on account of the general ignorance about
the human body, and the modern highly developed knowledge
of physiology. In this enterprise the most difficult task is to establish the first slender connecting link, after which with present-
day methods of research it would not be difficult to locate the
whole chain responsible for the phenomenon.

Resuming our description of the *nadis* we can safely identify
susumna with the spinal cord and its central canal, and *ida* and
pingala with the sympathetic and parasympathetic chains on the
left and right of it. *Pingala,* it is said, rises from the right testicle
and *ida* from the left one. This point needs clarification, since
the sympathetic and the parasympathetic systems innervate the
visceral organs and are also distributed in other parts of the body.
The preganglion neurons of the sympathetic chain rise from the
thoracic and lumber segments of the spinal cord, and those of
the parasympathetic from the brain and the sacral sections of the
cord. In the light of this fact the scrotum or the testicles cannot
be treated as the place of origin of these two *nadis*. The actual
position is that the whole area from the perineum to the navel

is thickly supplied with nerves from the central as well as the sympathetic and parasympathetic nervous systems. A large proportion of these nerves line the reproductive organs of both men and women. These chains of nerves are also joined by other nerves distributed over the right and left thigh, leg and foot. In an extended state of consciousness the nerve current moving through the chain of nerves designated as *pingala* distinctly appears to be hot and that moving through the *ida* cold. The perception of these two currents by introversion is one of the first developments that occurs on the awakening of *kundalini*.

The first center, or *muladhara cakra,* which plays a decisive part in the awakening, can be safely identified with the nerve junction between the anus and the root of the male organ. This is the most sensitive and the most important part in all the operations conducted by *kundalini* on awakening. We have purposely refrained from identifying the *nadis* and the *cakras* with this or that nerve or plexus, and will leave this task to the efforts of more competent investigators, who possess a thorough knowledge of the nervous system and the brain. The information we are recording is based on experience and inner observation. Thus it is impossible to be precise as to the exact nerve among the thousands or the exact spot which is involved in the operation. The specification of the nerves and their locations referred to here are tentative and should, therefore, be considered as mere approximations, subject to verification and study by other observers. This will avoid controversies and conflicts of the type that have occurred in the past. For the aim of this work is not to establish a new creed or to denigrate the existing ones, but to find a common basis and a common formula for them all. An error would be gratefully rectified, for it is by gradual expansion of his knowledge and correction of his mistakes that man has arrived at his present height.

In brief, it is a divine mechanism, which, with the awakening of the serpent power, springs to action to effect the liberation of the soul. The exponents of *kundalini* believe that the human body as a microcosm of the universe can duplicate the process of creation, maintenance, and dissolution of the Cosmos. They hold that so long as She lies coiled up above the *muladhara Cakra,* closing the aperture to *Brahman-rendra,* the embodied soul remains awake to the world, but when, with proper efforts, She is aroused and drawn upward to unite with Her spouse, Lord Shiva, in the *sahasrara,* the Yogi, now asleep in relation to the sensory world, awakens to the realization of his own divine nature. Her upward movement to the *Sahasrara* is, therefore, called *laya-karma,* or the process of dissolution, and Her descent back to *muladhara* is *Srsti-karma,* or the process of creation. For this reason Kundalini-Yoga is also called Laya-Yoga. One accomplished in this form of Yoga is thus said to be in possession of the power to create and destroy the world at will.

The idea that the serpent power is a limitless source of energy capable of investing the initiate, who has succeeded in arousing it, with entire command over the forces of nature, has no basis in reality, and is a product of the exaggerated accounts, contained in the ancient manuals, about the marvelous attributes of *kundalini.* These attributes aptly apply to the cosmic aspect of the creative energy, or *shakti,* but when applied to the individual the limitations that mark off the puny human creature from the almighty Cosmic Being must be applied to the individual aspect of *kundalini* as well. If it were not so, the very notion of "rousing Her from sleep" or "conducting Her to the *Sahasrara* or that "She should be led upward as a rider guides a mare with the reins", or that "She, the young widow, is to be despoiled by force" or that "With practice a Yogi becomes skilled in manipulating her" and other similar expressions used by ancient authors would be unthinkable. It is therefore obvious that the power alluded to is a potent life energy, normally in a dormant state, but capable of being activated with proper efforts directed to that end.

Considering the nature of the phenomenon to which it gives rise this energy can be compared with a powerful organic electric current of which, on the awakening of *kundalini,* the body becomes the generator. About this marvelous organic force the world of learning has no knowledge except that provided by Tantras and books on Hatha-Yoga. One part of this amazing energy, soaring high above the cloud of sensory knowledge, remains in perennial rapport with the pure, eternally bright sky of Universal Consciousness, while the other, rooted deep in the body, is governed by the laws of biology, depending for its activity on the nourishment provided by flesh and blood.

The fact that *ida* and *pingala* are said to arise from the left and right sides of the scrotum and the *susumna* from a place corresponding to the root of the generative organ, or that many of the practices of Hatha-Yoga, such as the position of the heels in the *siddhasana* and *padmasana* where they press upon the genital region or the repeated expansion and contraction of the anus by the manipulation of the anal sphincter muscle, advocated as a measure to facilitate the awakening, should not be understood to mean, as is sometimes supposed, that these practices are merely aimed to cause a stimulation of the sexual region and that the awakening of *kundalini* is no more than the reabsorption of the seminal fluid into the blood or its sublimation to cause ecstatic conditions of the mind. The actual fact is that the cerebro-spinal system, with the center of consciousness at the top and the reproductive region at the base, actuates in man the twofold purpose of the evolutionary as well as the reproductive mechanism. The three nerve channels, *ida, pingala,* and *susumna,* are the arteries of communication between the two extremities or poles. The confluence of *ida, pingala* and *susumna* at the level of the Ajna Cakra is known as Triveni. How deeply the concepts connected with *kundalini* have entered into the fundamentals of Hinduism is clear from the high degree of sanctity attached to the confluence of two or three sacred rivers, where millions bathe on certain auspicious occasions to wash away their sins or to gain liberation in symbolic imitation of the purgatorial office performed by *Shakti (kundalini)* on awakening. The solar and lunar *nadis* intersect with *susumna* at the various

Cakras. Finally at the Ajna Cakra, the place between the eyebrows, *kundalini* takes command of the mental functions, opening a new channel of perception, the sixth sense or the Third Eye, signifying the ascent to a higher step of the evolutionary ladder on the part of the successful initiate. From the Aina Cakra, *ida* and *pingala,* as is said, proceed to the right and left nostrils respectively, and the *susumna* enters the *sahasrara.*

If empiricism has not yet been able to locate the channel of communication between the two poles of this vital, two-pronged mechanism in the human body, the force of circumstantial evidence gathered from objective sources, even without subjective experience, would compel it to do so in the nearest future. The sympathetic and parasympathetic gangliated chains, the spinal cord, the reproductive system, and the brain are the greatest repositories of *prana,* or the organic vital essence in the body. This subtle organic medium is spread in every cell and part of the body, and functions as the connecting link between the superphysical cosmic *prana* and the flesh. The term *prana* repeatedly mentioned in the books on Kundalini-Yoga, usually refers to this subtle organic medium, the bridge between spirit and matter. In the living body this medium is manipulated by cosmic intelligence residing in the immaterial universal *prana or Pranashakti.* The marvelous functioning of the organic bodies, the cyclical memory of the genes, and the efficiency of the reproductive mechanisms, which stagger the intellect, depend on the superhuman intelligence present in the universal *prana,* the source of all life in the cosmos. Cosmic *prana* exists as a boundless universe of conscious energy, as an invisible self-generated all-pervasive current of intelligent electricity of illimitable power and unlimited speed, which, coming within the range of internal perception of the Awakened Man, brings into his consciousness other universes and other subtle energies that go into the making of this marvelous creation, whereof only an infinitesimal part is apprehended generally, by man with all his senses and intelligence.

The evolutionary-cum-reproductive mechanism in man functions in a manner in which the evolutionary aspect of it is completely shielded from the sphere of direct perception. While we are made acutely aware of the existence of the procreative activity of this mechanism by the constant presence of romantic and amorous thoughts in the mind and the behavior of the sexual organs, we have no awareness of a direct impact on our thoughts from the evolutionary aspect of it. Indirect evidence, complete almost to the point of being conclusive, is furnished by the so far imperfectly understood religious impulse and the unassuageable thirst for knowledge in the human mind, which, because of a hitherto fundamentally mechanistic conception of evolution, we have deplorably failed to explore and grasp. *Kundalini* is the key to the evolutionary mechanism. It is, therefore, but natural that it should be connected with and have influence over the spinal cord, the autonomic nervous system and the brain, for any stimulus to evolution to be effective must start from the cerebro-spinal directorate, and in order to be fruitful must have its closest cooperation and assistance at every step. Why it should be connected intimately with the reproductive system is abundantly clear from the very nature of Kundalini-Yoga, and the explanations furnished by its exponents. With the awakening of *kundalini* the successful initiate is in a position to utilize the tremendously potent *prana,* or organic life force, present in this region, for the important task of remodeling the brain and the nervous system to the point of evolutionary perfection, where man begins to approach the stature of a superman, adorned with new channels of perception and a Transcendent Consciousness, able to penetrate to the supersensible, subtle regions of the universe. This is the reason why Kundalini-Shakti has been revered by the ancients as a goddess and the deepest homage and worship offered to her.

The question posed at the beginning of this chapter as to when methods to manipulate this power center were practiced in India and were probably known to other countries also, why the knowledge of it is so scarce and the number of successful initiates so exceedingly small, provides in a way its own answer. Almost all of those who had this spiritual power center naturally active from birth, not being aware of the biological nature of the force at work in their bodies, usually attributed all manifestations and developments to divine favor, and where things went wrong to satanic or demonic influences, since from the very beginning all the phenomena proceeding from *kundalini* were attributed to super natural or divine agencies. In the case of those in whom the awakening occurred through prolonged effort, the Grace of God or the favor of the divine Shakti provided the answer to the weird manifestations and extraordinary occurrences that marked the course of the new development. That this has been so is fully corroborated by Tantras and other ancient works relating to *kundalini*. In dealing with *kundalini* we deal with a divine power center in man designed to lead him to a knowledge of his own immortal, superearthly nature by a process of sifting, purification, and remodeling, which, ordinarily might take hundreds, even thousands, of years. There must, therefore, be a certain state of preparedness and maturity, both mental and physical, in all those in whom the self-launched efforts terminate in success. Even with all these difficulties the number of those in whom the awakening, whether present from birth or resulting from practice, was successful in different parts of the world is surprisingly large. With the knowledge now available and the rapid rate of progress in almost all directions, the proportion of success is now likely to be a hundred times greater, if this divine quest is earnestly taken up by the luminaries of this age.

It hardly needs to be explained that for any system of Yoga or any spiritual effort to be successful, it is necessary that there should be a responsive agency in the body which the exercises can stimulate or influence in order to attain those states of consciousness in which mystical or any other spiritual experiences become possible. Without an agency of this kind and without some objective proof, establishing the existence of a superior mental state, beyond the normal capacity of the brain, as has been demonstrated by almost every genuine prophet, mystic, and saint, the validity of the experience in the case of those whose minds exhibit no other extraordinary development can be open to serious doubt. It is obvious that for any marked enhancement of the efficiency of the mind, beyond the normal limit, and for the exhibition of a more concentrated form of consciousness a biological readjustment of the brain would be absolutely necessary. Therefore every successful product of Yoga, religious effort, or occult practice must succeed in stimulating the device designed by nature to bring about the transformation, provided all the other factors combine to elicit a favorable response to such endeavor. This means that every effort which found access to supersensory states of consciousness must have, wittingly or unwittingly, made use of the evolutionary mechanism through its master key, *kundalini.*

The reason why so many conflicts and controversies arise between the adherents of different creeds, different systems of Yoga, or different schools of the occult is that the law underlying the manifestations has not been correctly understood. Can it be possible that the transcendent realm is so devoid of law that there is no uniform procedure to regulate the entry to it? Even such an idea is unthinkable. The prevailing belief that religious striving or Yoga in any form is undertaken to procure union with the divine, resulting in liberation from the bonds of flesh, is at the root of this misconception. The very concept of liberation connotes the idea of escape from the clutches of a painful world into the shielding arms of a merciful Deity waiting to receive the afflicted soul. This in turn implies that this desire in the heart of man to seek freedom from the world with its sorrows and burdens in the quest of the one Reality is inherent in the scheme of creation or, in other words, is in accordance with the will of the Creator. If this is conceded it would logically lead to the preposterous conclusion that all this stupendous universe has been brought into existence to place embodied souls deliberately in such a tormenting environment that, as soon as they possess the intelligence to understand their plight, they would fervently wish to be rid of it. Such a conception is entirely incompatible with the idea of a merciful Creator. The argument that bondage and emancipation are the fruits of *karma* and that the soul itself and not the Creator is responsible for it, does not provide a satisfactory answer to the problem. Conceding that karmic laws exist, do we know from which point they started? If not, how can we say where they will end? For all we know man might have to evolve to the stature of a god-like being in the millenniums he has still to live on this earth, and our efforts to interrupt this march of evolution by a premature withdrawal from the world might not be in accordance with the cosmic plan about the future destiny of mankind.

Just as every form of study stimulates the center of intelligence in the brain, and every form of artistic activity trains the muscles of the hand, the fingers, or the throat, leading to a better coordination between the organ and the mind, or as regular exercise tends to develop a particular group of muscles to which it is directed, so every form of religious exercise, Yoga, or occult practice tends to stir up *kundalini* which, in turn, by using a more potent *prana* and the precious substances, present in the reproductive secretions, starts an amazing process of remodeling designed to form a supersensory compartment in the brain—the ultimate object of the evolutionary impulse still active in man. The generally expressed view that in Raja-Yoga, Bakhti-Yoga, Karma-Yoga, or Jnana-Yoga, or in other forms of religious striving, *kundalini* is not awakened is not correct. It has already been discussed that for any religious effort to be successful it is necessary that it should press on some natural mechanism present in the body, failing which no change in consciousness can ever be possible. Swami Vivekananda voiced the same truth when he said, "Whenever there is any manifestation of what is ordinarily called supernatural power or wisdom there must have been a little current of *kundalini,* which found its way into the *susumna.*"

Unless there exists a natural arrangement already present in the brain by which its efficiency can be enhanced in the direction of supersensory or extrasensory perception no amount of mental training can lead to states of consciousness radically different from or superior to the normal pattern which is the common heritage of almost all mankind.

It cannot stand to reason that *kundalini* can be awakened only by violent and forcible methods as are embodied in the various schools of Hatha-Yoga. On the other hand, we can more realistically classify such methods as unnatural. If the existence of an evolutionary mechanism in the human body is conceded, it will also have to be admitted that its activity must be dependent on the stimuli of a certain type, coming either from the outside world or from the freely acting mind of the man himself. It will also have to be accepted that some of these stimuli must be more and some less effective in evoking a response, as is the case with every other organ in man, and that this power of responding and the mode of response must vary with the different individuals, as is the case with all other reflex systems in the body as well. This explains why some people are intensely religious, others moderately, others only slightly, and still others not at all, in the same way as some persons are very passionate, some moderately so, some only slightly and some so little that they seem to have no amorous feelings at all. In dealing with the evolutionary mechanism, as compared with the sexual process, we must remember the fact that, unlike the latter which has only the satisfaction of the procreative or erotic urge in view, the former expresses itself in the effort to find the solution to the mystery of existence and one's own being, the bedrock of religious inquiry, and the pursuit of knowledge to find the reasons for the natural phenomena urging one to raise oneself up to a position of power and well-being, the quest of the intellect. It is not, therefore, necessary that all people should be religious-minded. In those engrossed completely in the acquisition of knowledge, to the exclusion of religion, the evolutionary impulse is also active.

In every case of genuine mystical experience and spiritual illumination, the brain is fed by the superior, highly potent *prana,* or life force, poured by *kundalini* into it through the spinal duct after extraction from every part of the body. It is obvious that unless there is superior mental activity or the emergence of a higher consciousness to cause the phenomena, the whole experience dwindles down to a hallucination. It is also manifest that for a regular supernormal activity of the brain, a more potent type of energy to serve as fuel for it would be necessary. This is supplied by *kundalini.* The process of transformation, needed to arrange a regulated supply of this energy in accordance with the metabolic resources of the body, is a most complex and delicate operation, which remains in progress from the time the practice becomes effective. The aspirants to Yoga who believe that they can force the gates of heaven open with this or that method do not realize the stupendous nature of the task that they undertake. Whatever the method used for gaining transcendent knowledge or even occult powers and whatever the intensity of the effort the final arbiter of the award is *kundalini.* It is for this reason that from time immemorial the serpent power has been worshiped instinctively in countless forms and in numerous guises by almost all the people of the earth. Even those who place no reliance on religion and no faith in God, considering intellect to be the sole guide and architect of human fate, also pay homage to *kundalini* indirectly, for without the constant seepage of the Elixir of Life into the brain through the *susumna,* as an indispensable factor in the process of evolution, human thought could never have attained the towering heights it occupies at present.

9

The Harvest: Transcendence, Genius, and Psychic Powers

It has already been explained that *kundalini* is the spiritual as well as the biological base of all the phenomena connected with religion, the occult, and the supernatural. Whenever during the whole course of human history some man or woman exhibited uncanny powers which fell in the province of magic, witchcraft, augury, sorcery or mediumship and furnished conclusive evidence that the manifestations were genuine, in every case without exception, it signified the veiled activity of a slightly awake *kundalini*. In the same way, whenever any man or woman laid claim to prophethood, to direct communion with God or an Almighty Source of Intelligence and furnished irrefutable proof of supernormal faculties, higher moral standards, and mystical insight, it also, in every case, indicated a fully active *kundalini* that had found access to *sahasrara,* the highest center in the brain. Just as all variations, perversions, and distortions observed in the sexual behavior of individuals can only be attributed to the expression of the sex instinct, rooted in the reproductive mechanism, in the same way all the varied manifestations connected with religion and the supernatural have their origin in the dynamic spiritual power reservoir of *kundalini*.

In view of the fact that diverse conceptions about God, the

Soul, and the Beyond exist among people of different faiths, it is by no means an easy task to present the revolutionary ideas, embodied in this volume, so that they will coincide with the infinite mass of divergent and conflicting views held by the countless adherents of these various faiths. This task has become particularly difficult because of the fact that the existing literature on Yoga and *kundalini,* furnished by the modern popular treatises on the subject, presents a picture of both which often does not correspond to reality or the fundamental concept of Yoga as presented by the ancient adepts. Yoga and *kundalini* are interchangeable terms, for there is no Yoga and no union of the individual with Cosmic Consciousness unless *kundalini* is activated. The whole matter boils down to this: the human brain, as the result of evolution, has now the capacity to exhibit another kind of consciousness which can know itself or, in other words become conscious of consciousness, look beyond Space and Time. What is more surprising, instead of arriving at a conclusion by reasoning, as every normal mind does, it can dive into an Ocean of Knowledge in which all that is knowable is known, and all the problems awaiting solutions are solved. From this ocean droplets of fresh knowledge trickle down into normal consciousness, according to the degree of attunement with the brain, and it is these droplets of rare knowledge, not possible to recognize by empirical methods, which have always been honored as Revelation.

From the accounts of the transcendent state of consciousness, left by the mystics and seers of both the East and West, it is evident that the purpose of every form of religious striving, including Yoga, is to acquire a new state of Being in which one possesses new faculties higher than reason and thought. From the very beginning of recorded history every individual who achieved this state of Being invariably found it extremely difficult, even impossible, to describe his experience in terms comprehensible to his contemporaries. Even the most eloquent had to resort to parable, paradox, and metaphor in order to express the inexpressible experience. This difficulty still persists. From this it should not be inferred that we are expressing this difficulty as an avenue of escape from the responsibility of providing acceptable evidence for the objective nature of the phenomenon. But what we are saying is that just as we cannot describe the taste of salt to anyone who has never tasted it, so it is impossible through verbal description to convey even a remote idea of the transcendent state to those who have never experienced it.

Inexpressibility has always been a persistent feature of true mystical experience. "It is known to him," says the Kena Upanishad ((ii.2), "to whom it is unknown. It is unknown to those who (think they) know It well, and Known to those who do not know." How the knower of *Brahman* expresses his own bewilderment at the experience is described in the verse preceding it: "I do not think I know (*Brahman*) well enough: Not that I do not know: I know and do not know as well. He amongst us who understands that utterance: 'Not that I do not know, I know and I do not know as well,' knows that (*Brahman*)." Those who are filled with an insatiable desire to have a vision of God or to have access to higher planes of consciousness are only motivated by promptings from the evolutionary center in the brain to overstep the bounds of human consciousness. In the case of mystics and seers in the past, the transition was sometimes sudden. This was achieved by intense meditation, burning desire, and austerity, and the higher center began to function abruptly causing, as it were, an explosion in consciousness, leaving the initiate shaken and breathless with the vision of a stupendous and entirely unexpected transformation within himself. It is no wonder that the supramental, living Reality that now unfolded in the consciousness of the visionary was regarded as the Supreme Ruler, Creator, or the Author of the universe.

The most pressing need of our age is to widen the inner horizons of consciousness. This widening is necessary to counterbalance the staggering effect on the intellect caused by the present-day enormously increased knowledge of the universe, which relegates the earth, the solar system, and even man, to a state of utter insignificance in a gigantic whole. This sense of irrelevance and isolation may not be so pronounced in the case of those who hold dominating positions in any sphere of human activity: in science, philosophy, art, industry, finance, politics, sports, and the like, but its effect on the more intelligent and more sensitive among the masses is often devastating. The explosive situation of the world today is the direct outcome of the outer and inner imbalance. The enormous increase in the number of drug addicts, the march of millions toward an unbridled, chaotic life in the fruitless effort to gain inner peace, the rush toward Yoga and other occult practices in order to experience the numinous, the constant scenes of disorder and destruction, violence, war, revolutions, and riots in an age when technology has brought formerly undreamed-of amenities within the grasp of every man, constitute a phenomenon about which no explanation in terms of current knowledge is possible. In actual fact, the real reason for this uncontrollable situation is that with the growing complexity and widening of the outer world a corresponding enlargement of the inner horizons is also necessary to save man from being completely crushed under the ponderous load of his own creation.

The development of mystical insight that grants to the over-awed intellect a glimpse of the nature of the inner Self cannot, therefore, be considered either a luxury, a hobby, or a fancy with respect to those who pursue the goal, but as an unavoidable necessity for the survival of a sane and sober humanity. It is incredible that the evolutionary purpose served by the mystical impulse has not been recognized even by learned explanations, comparable to those which primitive minds offered for the mysterious phenomena of nature. The transporting effect of light and color, of gems, of beautiful colored glass, of superb painting, sculpture, and music becomes suspect since it is considered to be an aid to hallucinatory experience, to an excursion into "the mind's antipodes". On the contrary these objects serve to remind the ego-consciousness of the marvelous transformation that is occurring in its depths, of the gradually developing wondrous state of Being which, when one looks inward, will appear lustrous as "an isle of gems," glowing as a "mountain of burnished gold," vast as the ocean, more alluring to the sense of sight, touch, hearing, taste, and smell than all the most enchanting works of art, music, and all the most delicious aromas, viands, and bodily sensations put together. On the wings of destiny every member of the human race is soaring inwardly toward a state of splendor, harmony, and peace that has no parallel in the universe we observe. The transporting effect of meditation on divine objects, of prayer, of magnificent places of worship, the solemn atmosphere in shrines, the touching life stories of prophets and saints, the profound utterances of sages and seers lie in their appeal to the evolutionary instinct which is drawing man toward a higher dimension of consciousness, toward a glorious inner universe in which all his uncorrupted ambitions, aspirations, and ideals will find fulfillment.

Can there be any doubt that these instances portray a condition of inner transformation. The ego-consciousness now in contact with the Universe of Life, with the Ocean of which she is but a droplet, feels one with It and yet overawed by the Majesty treats it as Something beyond and above it. Even in the normal state, the ultimate nature of the world we apprehend is something mysterious. It is a picture presented to us by our senses and the intellect. Every species of fish, reptile, bird, and animal perceives a different, though not a radically different, world. The mysterious senses of ants, bees, bats, dogs, migratory birds, and the like are incomprehensible to us because the world is presented to each in a different way so that certain things that are entirely beyond the realm of our cognition are a normal feature of their perception. We see and we know what we are permitted to see and know by our mind, which is conditioned by the capacity of the brain. Problems of life and death or the origin and the purpose of the universe do not torment the animal. Even in the human sphere these problems have different values and different degrees of urgency for different people. What modern psychology fails to recognize is the fact that different people are at different levels of the evolutionary ascent, and that the human brain is still in a state of transition. So long as this cardinal fact is not accorded due recognition, no systematic study of mind is possible.

Problems of life and death, the here and the hereafter assume a greater urgency for those who are spiritually oriented. For some they become the most dominating influence in shaping the course of life. Those endowed with this type of thirst not infrequently change from one school of discipline to another and read avidly one book after another to discover a way to assuage this thirst without meeting any success. There is a strong reason for the disappointments often encountered by people of this class in their search. The thirst is the pointer to a certain target and the pole star guiding the mind toward a certain altered condition of consciousness in which the problem, never arising in the animal mind but tormentingly pursuing man at every step, finding a complete answer, then ceases to oppress. The problem arises in the human mind because the intellect is constituted in this way, and as long as it does not come across a mode of apprehension superior to its own it can never feel satisfied and never come to rest. With the enhancement of the intellect, unless there is degeneration, the problem becomes more pressing. This is actually what has happened in our time. Unless the knower in man overreaches the senses and the intellect and asserts its own importance and position of power in relation to the stupendous, mighty world the human mind can know no peace. This is the reason why those thirsty for knowledge of the Self are acutely conscious of disappointments and failures, for until the transition is complete and the intellect pacified with the vision, the mind continues to fret.

All that we are and all that we know are circumscribed by the capacity of the knower in us. The world appears gigantic and monstrous because we identify ourselves completely with the body and measure the vastness of the universe by its size. Viewed apart from the body, unconditioned by the mind and intellect, the knower transcends the known, for the latter can never exceed the power of comprehension of the former and must always remain subservient to its capacity. The moment transcendence occurs, the objective universe loses its importance as well as its magnitude. This is what Jacob Boehme tries to express, colored of course with ingrained theistic ideas, when he says: "In one quarter of an hour I saw and knew more than if I had been many years together at a University. For I saw and knew the being of all things, The Byss and the Abyss and the eternal generation of the holy Trinity, the descent and origin of the world and of all creatures through the divine wisdom. I knew and saw in myself all the three worlds, the external and visible world of a procreation or external birth from both the internal and spiritual worlds; and I saw and knew the whole working essence, in evil and in good, and the origin of existence; and likewise how the fruitful bearing womb of eternity was brought forth. So that I did not only greatly wonder at it, but did also exceedingly rejoice, albeit I could very hardly apprehend the same in my external man and set it down with the pen. For I had a thorough view of the universe as in a chaos, wherein all things are couched and wrapt up, but it was impossible for me to explicate the same."*

The same idea of transcendence is expressed in the Rig-Veda (x.90.1-3) in these words: ". . . He is the all-pervading Being manifesting himself as all things. He has innumerable heads, eyes and feet. It is He that has encompassed the whole universe, and it is He again who transcends it. . . . "That Being is this whole cosmos, all that was and all that will be. He manifests Himself in the form of the universe. He is also the lord and giver of immortality. . . . So vast is His glory; but He, the universal Being, is greater than all that. The manifested world forms but a small portion of His being; in main He is unmanifest and

* *The Three Principles of the Divine Essence*, Jacob Boehme; K. W. Schiebler, Leipzig, 1922.

immortal." Taittiriya Āranyaka (x.11) presents the same view thus: "He transcends the whole world, and also manifests Himself as the whole world. He is the eternal Being, the support of all, the remover of evil. The existence of the whole world depends on Him. He is the master of the world, the supreme Self, the eternal, the permanent good, the changeless, the Cosmic Being, the great goal of knowledge, the Self of the universe and the supreme refuge. . . ." The transformed consciousness, cognizant now of its infinite nature, immeasurably superior to the universe known by the senses, which continues to abide in its finite form, transcends and overshadows it, calming the unrest of the intellect convinced now beyond the least shadow of a doubt that the All-Pervading Knower and not the conditioned Known is the substratum of the universe.

Through divine dispensation, for some purpose which only the future can disclose, this frail, human creature, with a limited span of life, which some birds, fishes, and other lowly creatures exceed, with a body so delicate that even one blow at a vulnerable spot is sufficient to cause death, and a mind and memory so restricted that it cannot grasp more than an infinitesimal fraction of the cosmos, by the favor of Destiny with but a slight alteration in the vital energy feeding the brain, overcoming the limitations imposed by the senses, can soar to a state of Existence where the ruthless, colossal world becomes a fleeting shadow and he the Effulgent Sun. Death and fear then lose their hold, for what can harm the Ocean of Everlasting Life beyond the farthest reach of any profane material influence? It is in this sense of achieving a State of Consciousness, characterized by immortality and infinitude that it is said in the ancient works on Kundalini-Yoga that the accomplished Sadhka can create, preserve, and destroy the world at will. The underlying idea is that in the transcendent state which he attains with full lucidity, the world image which first dominated his unreal, sense-bound consciousness, recedes into insignificance.

Transcendence is as far removed from the hallucinatory states of mind brought about by drugs, autohypnosis, autointoxication, and changes in body chemistry as the consciousness of absolute power and incomparable dignity in an anointed king, ruling over a vast empire, is removed from the delusive state of a psychotic who, disorderly and unkempt, raves at the top of his voice about his kingdom and his court. The general ignorance prevailing among the people, including even scholars, about the real nature of the beatific state is at the root of the present confusion, resulting in the waste of precious lives of those who fall prey to the delusion that drugs and other artificial methods can lead to the exalted state in which man for the first time steps over the rigid boundaries of mortal consciousness. It is not merely a change in the brilliance of colors of the objects seen, nor alteration or distortion in their shape, nor the revelation of a new significance in them, nor the transitory awareness of a new insight that is decisive in determining the genuineness of a mystical experience, but the change that occurs in the Fount of personality or, in other words, in the Knower, which is the distinguishing feature of the phenomenon. The Knower undergoes a complete metamorphosis; from a drop he becomes an ocean and from a point of awareness an infinite circle of sovereign consciousness.

Shankaracarya in Vivekacudamani (389 and 394) expresses the state of transcendence in these words: "The Self is within, and the Self is without, the Self is before and the Self is behind, the Self is in the south, and the Self is in the north; the Self likewise is above as below . . . . What is the use of dilating on this subject? The Jiva (embodied consciousness) is no other than *Brahman* (Universal Consciousness), this whole extended universe is *Brahman* Itself, the Shruti inculcates the *Brahman* without a Second, and it is an indubitable fact that people of enlightened minds who know their identity with *Brahman* and have given up their connection with the objective world, live palpably united with *Brahman* as Eternal Knowledge and Bliss." The Knower, surpassing now both the material universe and the world of thought, or, in other words, merging in itself the process of knowing and the known, assumes an aspect which no language can express and no intelligence grasp. "You cannot see the seer of sight," says the *Brhadaranyaka Upanishad* (3.4.2.). "You cannot hear the hearer of hearing, you cannot think the thinker of thought, you cannot know the knower of knowledge. This is your self that is within all. Everything besides this is perishable." The same idea of the incomprehensibility of the eternal, unconditioned Knower is again expressed in the same Upanishad (3.8.1) in these words: "He is never seen but is the Seer; He is never heard, but is the Hearer; He is never thought, but is the Thinker; He is never known, but is the Knower. There is no other seer than He, there is no other hearer than He, there is no other thinker than He, there is no other knower than He. He is the Inner Controller—your own self and immortal. All else but Him is perishable."

A radical transformation in the foundations of a man's personality, as comes to pass in the case of an accomplished Yogi, is actually a transformation in the nature of the Knower who is now in a position to perceive both the inner and the outer worlds. Such an alteration cannot occur without changing the whole mental structure of a man. This is exactly what this volume is intended to pinpoint and to prove. The fact that people in general are not properly educated about the real nature of the metamorphosis brought about by Yoga is at the root of the present-day flood of faulty literature on the subject from the pens of authors lacking completely in experience of the mystical state. This has done and is doing grave harm by disseminating wrong and sometimes even dangerous information about an undertaking requiring expert guidance and extreme care at every step. The other evil that has resulted from this ignorance is that false prophets and sham Gurus have sprung up and dominate the stage everywhere, especially in the West, reducing this venerable system of spiritual discipline to a farce, and in this way doing great disservice to a cause which in the present critical situation of the world is of paramount importance.

The ancient authors, especially those writing on Kundalini-

Yoga, have made no secret of the divine attributes (*vibhutis*) and miraculous powers (*siddhis*) that automatically develop in one who attains perfection in Yoga. Patanjali, in his Yoga-Sutras, has devoted one full chapter of his book to the discussion of supernatural powers (*siddhis*). There is another aspect, even more important and fascinating, on which it is necessary to dwell here. If purely from the aspect of commonsense we soberly consider the idea of a metamorphosis of consciousness, involving a change from a human to a transhuman level, would it not be but rational to suppose that such a radical change in order to be genuine, and not merely an illusion, must be attended by other attributes of mind and intellect that are not found as a normal feature in human beings? It would be inaccurate to maintain that one who comes in contact with a Source of Infinite Intelligence in his ecstasies and visions would continue to have the same mental caliber afterward as he had before such an experience. His mental capacity and intellectual stature must show an enormous improvement and surpass in some respects, at least, the highest intellects of the time. It was primarily on account of the fact that in their power of expression and intellectual endowments the prophets and seers of the past towered head and shoulders over their contemporaries that they were able to win the respect and admiration of multitudes who accepted their teachings.

While the ancient masters have paid due attention to this aspect of Yoga and, in their writings, plainly brought out the fact that success in the enterprise is attended by remarkable increase in intellectual powers and by the development of literary talents and gifts, the modern authors have maintained an unaccountable silence over this important issue. Most of them have lavishly dwelt on the higher states of consciousness and miraculous powers but one notable achievement (the development of genius) has been, for some reason, completely ignored. One reason for this can be that they did not attach any importance to the repeated assertions made in the ancient works, treating them as mere euphemisms, and the other that the idea was so far from their minds that they failed to grasp the significance of these assertions though, in the course of their study, they must have come across them repeatedly. The omission appears incredible considering the emphasis that the ancient authors have laid on this development. To the question of the present-day scholar, the development of enhanced intellectual powers and genius in one not endowed with them from birth is impossible because of the hereditary factors involved, depending on the nature of the genes. It is sufficient to say at this place that it is precisely in this aspect of Yoga that the possibility of objective demonstration lies in its most striking form.

It is evident (see also Appendix, pp. 204 to 207) that from Vedic times, persisting through the Upanishads, and coming down almost to our own day, there has always existed a strong belief that with the arousal of a normally dormant divine energy in him, a man of common clay can be transformed into an intellectual prodigy; an invincible giant in polemics, a most eloquent speaker and a poet whose "random talk even will take the form of poetry." Making every allowance for exaggeration, even if a fraction of the affirmations of ancient authors are accepted as correct, it discloses a tremendous possibility hidden in Yoga about which not only the masses but even the learned are entirely in the dark at present. There is every likelihood, considering the vein of extreme devotion and utter surrender to the divine *shakti (kundalini)* permeating the ancient treatises on the subject, particularly those in verse, that many of the authors themselves were the recipients of the favor and had witnessed the marvelous transformation in themselves. There is hardly any well-known Yoga saint in India who has not left a precious legacy of a priceless spiritual document in beautiful verse. To the seeker who practices Yoga to gain visionary experience or to develop psychic talents, this aspect of the discipline might not seem to be of any particular worth, but, considered from a pragmatic point of view, there is no side as useful for the enlighten-

ment of the seekers and as precious for a scientific exploration of
the possibilities, latent in it, as this.

If mystical experience of the genuine kind, whether brought
about by Yoga or any other form of religious discipline, represents a real unfolding of the spirit, or a vision of God, it must
be attended by a blossoming of the mental fabric of the individual as well. If the blossoming does not occur and the mystic
merely revels in his own enrapturing visions without possessing
the ability to communicate his experiences in order to share
them with the world, the whole achievement is reduced to the
level of a fantasy or a daydream which, however pleasant it may
be for the daydreamer, has no meaning or importance for others.
Spiritual ideals and institutional religions possess a meaning and
a value for mankind because the gifted individuals who popular-
ized or founded them possessed in ample measure the talent to
express their ideas and experiences in a manner that touched
the heart and appealed to the intellect of their contemporaries.
The idea common to the devout that their religion is revealed
and God-ordained has a profound bearing on our present theme.
That the scriptures have emanated from God, the Fountainhead
of all knowledge and wisdom, conveys indirectly the highest
tribute to the intellectual caliber of those who served as channels
for the dissemination of the Revealed Teachings. From whatever
aspect we examine it, the conclusion is irresistible that intellectual
efflorescence is and should be an inseparable companion to spiritual enrichment.

The close connection between these two highest expressions of
the human mind has, in its turn, a profound significance in relation to the present explosive situation of the world. Intellectual
advancement must accompany spiritual growth. If the former
occurs without a corresponding spiritual development it is a
sign that the growth is one-sided and, therefore, abnormal, an
indication that something is radically wrong with the society and
a warning that danger lies ahead if the harmony is not restored.
As spiritual perfection connotes the manifestation of a higher

human personality that has crossed beyond the limit, where common mortals come to a halt, it necessarily implies an all-round development in the mental capacity of the perfected person. It would be an anomaly if those who attain a lofty stature spiritually continue to be pygmies in intellect. The ancient authors, therefore, give expression to a very plain truth when they associate enhancement in intellectual acumen with spiritual perfection. While for the ancient this synchronous development of the two did not involve any factor antagonistic to the accepted ideas of the age, the present position is not as favorable for the modern intellectual. The transition from a state of mediocrity to a position of intellectual eminence in the light of the beliefs current in this age is for the average person an impossibility, and the concept that Yoga, or any other form of spiritual discipline, provides a sure way to its achievement is likely to be regarded with disbelief and even ridicule.

It is precisely because the idea is so unacceptable to the modern scholar, steeped in the materialistic trends of the time, that this aspect of Yoga has a profound significance for our age. That it is possible for one to blossom into a Samkara, a Michaelangelo, a Hafiz, a Newton, Vyasa, a Plato, or an Einstein, with a certain kind of psycho-physiological discipline, is an idea so novel and so full of undreamed-of possibilities in this age of science that it outweighs all other present-day concepts by its importance and the promises it holds. Even if this possibility is admitted, there is little chance for any vast improvement of the world, since the phenomenon is so rare and the chances of a successful termination of the practice are so remote that the radical transformation wrought in the whole of mankind by a few scores of men of genius in this period of history is a sufficient guarantee that even a few transformed adepts in this or in any future age cannot but prove a most valuable asset to mankind. This is not all. There is every chance that once the possibility is empirically demonstrated and the law is established, the modern high degree of advance in the knowledge of psychology, therapy and physiology would prove of inestimable value in improving the efficiency of the disciplines and minimizing the risks. The day is not distant, once the biological intricacies connected with the awakening of *kundalini* are known, when this divine enterprise will provide the most contested and most sought-after trophy for the luminaries of the time.

We live in an age of surprises. At the same time, we experience the horror of man-caused calamities. But no surprise has been so great as will take place when this law is empirically demonstrated, and no calamity has been so devastating as might befall if, in the present stage of technological development, the law is still ignored. The development of the human brain and the intellect is an unavoidable consequence of evolution, but without spiritual discipline and enlightenment the results can not only be unwholesome but also fatally poisonous. The scope of this volume does not permit us to dwell on the *kali* aspect of *kundalini*, the punitive phase when for the purpose of destruction, She, in a malignant form, is awake from birth in a demagogue or a dictator. The effort has been made here to bring into focus the vital issues involved in a study of *kundalini* and the imperative need for controlled genius in the present age. "With its roots above and branches below they speak of the eternal Asvattha tree," says the Bhagavad-Gita (xv.1). "Whose leaves are the Vedas; he who knows this is a knower of the Vedas." The Asvattha tree is the evolving phenomenal world. The impulse toward evolution comes from the root, that is, from the unmanifested Eternal Intelligence acting through cosmic *prana,* but for its correct translation and the proper adjustment of life, both individual and collective, to the needs of this impulse, knowledge of the Vedas, that is, both temporal and divine knowledge, is necessary. In other words, it is essential in order to ensure smooth progress and safety on the hazardous path of evolution that man should not only be possessed of temporal knowledge but should also know the laws that rule his spiritual growth. This is why *gayatri mantra* (the knowledge of *kundalini*) is said to be the quintessence of the Vedas.

How poor the current picture is of the lofty science of Yoga, especially in the West, can be observed from the fact that one dressing himself in a certain peculiar way, or one who can stand on his head for a few minutes, or one who, when he touches you, exhales a certain perfume, or one who sits calm and silent in a certain posture for prolonged spells is regarded as a Yogi. There is not the least inquiry as to the way by which such a person has transcended the normal mental state of an intelligent man. If there has been no such crossing of the boundary line, it means that Yoga has not been accomplished and, however learned or calm or self-controlled or physically healthy or agile a man might be, he is still as far from the consummation of Yoga as any other average individual. Even the awakening of *kundalini*, unattended by a metamorphosis of consciousness to the point of transcendence, does not make one aware of the supersensory realms. One in whom such an awakening occurs may display some psychic gifts, but in other respects he rises no higher than a common medium or sensitive. For real transformation or, in other words, for the fruition of Yoga one must be in rapport with higher planes of existence and have access to Supernal Wisdom which flows from the truly enlightened even as fragrance exudes from a blooming rose.

The picture of the accomplished Yogi, presented by the ancient authors, though exaggerated and distorted here and there, has a solid core of truth so alluring and so precious, for both the individual and the race, that no other human undertaking is comparable to it. The moment transcendence occurs, the aspirant blossoms into a genius of a high order. Simultaneously other windows in the mind open and, to his unbounded surprise and joy, he finds himself in possession of channels of communication which, acting independently of the senses, can bring to him knowledge of events, occurring at a distance, as also visions of the past and future. His utterances may become prophetic (*vaksiddhi*) and he may acquire the healing touch.

The one important lesson, especially relevant to this age, which Yoga imparts is that the stupendous universe we live in is but a

compartment in a mammoth edifice of which the other compartments are not perceptible to our senses. The other numerous
compartments might be as vast or even vaster than the one discernible to us to the farthest limits of space, and they all might
be interpenetrating or overlapping each other without the inhabitants of one being aware of the proximity of the other. Just
as some pictures show the face of one person from one side and
that of another from the other, and of a third when viewed from
the front, in the same way the universe, perceptible to our senses
might be multifaced, that is, might have innumerable facets,
presenting as it were a different form to each separate level of
consciousness, appearing as an objective reality to a normal
human mind and as a vanished dream to one in *turiya*. It is also
possible that there might be innumerable other forms of life on
different planes of consciousness, operating with different types
of sensitive equipment. In the culminating state of Yoga we
merely shift from one plane of consciousness to another.

When this happens the world normally visible to us loses its
grip on the mind. It is in this sense that the Upanishads compare
it to a dream or to a rope imagined to be a snake or a mirage
mistaken for an oasis. The actual fact is that the world is not a
myth or a pure illusion, but though real in one dimension of
consciousness, becomes a shadow or vanishes altogether in the
other. The classification of human consciousness into three states
of waking, dream, and dreamless slumber, made by the ancient
seers of India is to bring into relief the fourth state, *turiya*, which
includes in it all the three states and yet is above and beyond
them, or, in other words, which represents another dimension
of consciousness in which the material world loses its objectivity
for the Yogi, now in direct contact with other planes of Being.
This is how Sankaracarya expresses these variations in consciousness in the beginning of his commentary on the Mandukya Upanishad: "I bow to that *Brahman,* which, after having enjoyed (during the waking state) all gross objects by pervading the entire
universe with the omnipresent rays of Its immutable Conscious-

ness, embracing the entire variety of movable and immovable objects; which, again, after having digested, as it were—that is to say, experienced within (in the dream state)—all the variety of objects produced by desires and brought into existence by the mind, enjoys bliss in deep sleep and makes us experience that bliss through *maya*; which further is designated in terms of *maya* as the fourth (*turiya*), and which is supreme, immortal and changeless."

Entrance into *turiya* is entrance into a dimension of consciousness, above the normal human level. This does not make the world, perceptible at the human level, unreal or illusory in the least. To say so would be to deny the reality of *turiya* also, for it is only when viewed from the human aspect that the significance of *turiya* can be understood. If there were no human level of consciousness there would be no *turiya* either. As such it is fallacious to hold that for one who has attained the knowledge of *Brahman* in *turiya,* the world should cease to hold any value or importance. In actual fact, a contrary view would be more sensible and accurate. As it is in the world that our bodies and minds are nourished and, again, as it is because of the world that the higher state of consciousness, experienced in *samadhi* or *turiya,* is attained, it naturally devolves as a duty on one who has tasted the Supreme Bliss of this indescribable state to exert himself to the utmost to help others to reach the same summit in order to repay the debt he owes to the world and to the countless people of the world whose labor, directly or indirectly, contributed in innumerable ways to his existence, maintenance and, finally, to the achievement that brought him such glory and joy. In a law-bound Creation it is obvious that this higher plane of consciousness cannot be a prize, reserved for a few; but what we have failed to recognize so far, is that it must be a summit which every member of the race is destined to reach one day. Those who climb to it first, acting as pioneers, must guide others on the steep ascent until the task is accomplished, and the whole caravan arrives safely at the top.

There was a day when the earth was considered to be the center
of the universe, around which the sun, the moon, and the stars
obediently revolved. Further investigation has revealed an altogether different picture of the cosmos and, far from being the
center of creation, the earth, it has now been established, holds
a very insignificant position in a gigantic host. Is it not reasonable
to suppose that what applies to the outer universe might be true
of the inner one also and that the conception that *turiya* is the
highest state of existence and the last summit of consciousness
might be as illusory as was the notion that the earth is the primary center of all existence? This faulty conception might have
been based on the equally erroneous idea that man is the cream
of all creation, a clearcut symptom of arrogance and self-conceit,
similar to that which led ancient kings to claim a divine origin
for themselves. To hold that attainment to superconsciousness
entitles one to claim identity with the Creator or *Brahman* is
tantamount to bringing the Almighty First Cause down to the
level of puny man or raising this frail creature to the stature of
the All-powerful Ruler of the cosmos, both unmistakable symptoms of self-adulation and pride. We have not yet been able to
establish, to the satisfaction of all sections of humanity, the
reality of transcendent states of consciousness, and the accounts
of those who claim to have attained it are so varied and divergent
that it is not surprising that doubts are raised about the validity
of the whole phenomenon in the minds of many people. To dismiss these genuine doubts as mere delusion is not reasonable on
the part of those who believe in its reality and, if such an attitude
is adopted by one who has attained Transcendence, it reveals
the continued existence in his enlightened mind of that most
stubborn of human frailities: pride.

"In the same way as the unwise act with attachment," says the
Bhagavad-Gita (3.25 and 26), "so should the wise act without
attachment for the guidance of the world . . . (and) let not the
wise unsettle the understanding of the ignorant, attached to
action, but acting himself with equipoise should engage them in

action also." In the present state of our knowledge when Transcendence is still an unverified and disputed phenomenon, and the territory is still as foreign to the normal mind as the landscape of an unseen planet, would it not be presumptuous on the part of one who has entered a higher plane of consciousness to jump to conclusions about the Ultimate, when he himself has not made sure that he has touched the peak of human evolution and that there is no other summit higher than the one he has reached? There can be no more potent factor to humble a man of intelligence and to deflate his pride than the contemplation of the starry firmament at night and the realization of his own utterly insignificant position in the innumerable host of colossal suns which he perceives. Similarly, there is no more potent factor to humble the pride of an Awakened man than the infinitely vaster dimensions of the universe of consciousness he glimpses within. The most sensible thing for both the intellectual and the man of vision, in the present state of our knowledge, is to exchange ideas in order to identify the basic factors underlying all genuine spiritual experience and then to devise methods to establish the validity of the phenomenon beyond doubt and dispute.

The investigation has to be undertaken in all humility because, in approaching the supersensible, man for the first time comes in conscious contact with Intelligent Forces that are not amenable to mortal control. What those engaged in this investigation must always keep before their minds is the indisputable fact that their very existence, about which they know almost nothing, depends entirely on the benign disposition of these Intelligent Forces. When benignly disposed *kundalini* can transform a commonplace, humble man into a seer, a prophet, an intellectual giant, or a world teacher, with extraordinary talents and supernormal gifts, but approached arrogantly or with impure motives, the same Energy, malignantly disposed, can change the most clever man into a gibbering maniac in such a dreadful state of self-torture that death would be merciful in comparison. During the last approximately one hundred years, in spite of repeated attempts made by competent investigators, including prominent men of science, to place supernormal phenomena on a scientific footing, the success achieved has been almost negligible and the world is still torn by doubts about this momentous issue, close to the heart of every human being. The reason for it lies in the fact that approach to Divinity for enlightenment has to be made in a different spirit and in a way other than that adopted for the investigation of physical phenomena. The sphere of the spirit has been carefully shielded by nature from the prying eyes of the curious, and only those few who pass the scrutiny of the Cosmic Forces that guard access to the Higher Planes of Consciousness, are allowed to pass through. These screening devices are present in the human brain, and are acted upon by the cosmic *prana* in the same way as it acts on the genes. It is because access to the spiritual kingdom is so closely guarded that the investigation of psychic phenomena, carried on for the past several decades, has not been decisive in solving the riddle or even in furnishing conclusive evidence this way or that. The believers continue to believe, but the skeptics are still unconvinced about the independent and deathless nature of the spirit.

In their intellectual stature, the leading thinkers of the race have almost touched the threshold of the divine, but, for access, a high degree of perfection in all the three components of personality, mental, moral, and physical, is necessary before the doors will swing open. In support of our assertion it is enough to point out that in every system of Yoga development of all three aspects of personality is invariably kept in view. "The Self is not attained by one devoid of strength," says the Mundaka Upanishad (3.2.4), "nor through delusion, nor through austerity devoid of system; But the Self of that Knower, who strives through these means enters into the abode that is *Brahman.*" The mighty problem of life and death is the bait, dangled tantalizingly by nature before the human mind, to draw man toward a higher state of consciousness. Those whose minds treat this problem as the first priority are the ones who accept Yoga or other forms of spiritual discipline